Still Above Ground: My Badass Battle with Cancer

Jeri Kroll

BLUE BOAT BOOKS

Ipswich, Massachusetts

Still Above Ground

COPYRIGHT © 2020 BY **JERI KROLL**

All rights reserved. No part of this publication may be reproduced, distributed or transmitted in any form or by any means, without prior written permission.

Blue Boat Books
46 Argilla Road
Ipswich, Massachusetts/USA 01983
krolljeri@gmail.com

Publisher's Note: This work is autobiographical. Although the author and publisher have made every effort to ensure that the information in this book was correct at press time, the author and publisher do not assume and hereby disclaim any liability to any party for any loss, damage, or disruption caused by errors or omissions, whether such errors or omissions result from negligence, accident, or any other cause.

Book Layout © 2017 BookDesignTemplates.com

Cover Design by Patch Kroll

Still Above Ground/Jeri Kroll. -- 1st ed.
ISBN 978-1-7320804-2-3

Jeri Kroll

DEDICATED TO

The Staff at Lahey Healthcare

Laura Jett, MD
Primary Care Physician

Andrew Wiechert, MD
Caroline Nitschmann, MD
Gynecologic Oncologists

Andrea Bertram Mckee, MD
Radiation Oncologist

The nurses, technicians, other medical personnel, social workers, receptionists and volunteers at:

The Sophia Gordon Cancer Center
Burlington, Massachusetts
Peabody, Massachusetts

You are all truly awesome.

"She stood in the storm, and when the wind did not blow her way, she adjusted her sails."
Elizabeth Edwards
American attorney, author
Resilience and the Burdens and Gifts of Facing Life's Adversities
Breast cancer

"Love and laughter are two of the more important universal cancer treatments on the planet. Overdose on them."
Tanya Masse
Canadian writer
Stripping Away the Insanity of Life and Parenthood

"Don't look back, you're not going that way."
Anonymous

Jeri Kroll

Introduction

When I was first diagnosed with cancer, even when I thought it was only going to be a matter of surgery, I started keeping a diary. I was hoping it would amount to a few entries about my operation which would be quite boring and that at some point, I'd discard the wannabe journal. As it turns out I now have 10 months' worth of entries. I did not record an entry every day as one might in a "Dear Diary" type journal. Many days I didn't have the energy to write much other than "Spent the day in the bathroom" or "Today is Friday - I think." Nobody wants to read that type of daily drivel, myself included.

Three items of note:
1. As I re-read and edited the journal in preparation for publishing, I felt compelled at times to add a few thoughts. In an effort to remain true to the purpose of documenting the journey, text added later appears in [*brackets and italicized text*].

2. A word about the title which I arrived at early on. I liked the phrase "still above ground" – assuming I still am. I struggled with the word "badass" because, as you will see, I'm really not. However, the word is kind of "in" right now and "badass battle" has an alliterative advantage. A more accurate title would be Still Above Ground: One Wimpy Bitch's Battle with Cancer. The deciding factor was that given a choice, I'd pick up a book describing the author as a "badass battler" rather than

as a "wimpy bitch." I suppose in the end the reader can decide which is more accurate.

3. My purpose in sharing my journal is to encourage others traveling down a similar path. In assessing the manuscript as a whole, however, it occurs to me that the reader might be horrified rather than comforted! The fact is cancer isn't pretty. Cancer isn't funny. Cancer isn't fun. But there is humor to be found along the way and with the support of others and the ability to laugh at ourselves cancer won't defeat, demoralize or diminish us.

Jeri Kroll

Preface

To provide the basic background of this journal the following is a summary of my cancer journey.

I was diagnosed with endometrial cancer in October 2018. What started out as an annual physical and a minor complaint about acid reflux led to about eight months of multiple ultrasounds, MRIs, CAT scans, blood tests, two endoscopies, a hysteroscopy, a colonoscopy and for good measure, pun intended, we squeezed in a mammogram. When all was said and done the doctors felt this was an early diagnosis so that a hysterectomy would take care of it. I had surgery on October 22nd removing the uterus, the ovaries (one with a cyst), a large fibroid tumor and a couple of lymph nodes. These organs and growths apparently and unfairly do not weigh anything.

The afternoon following the hysterectomy the surgeon told me and my partner, Jodi, that everything looked good but of course they would biopsy the tissue that was removed. A week later I got "the call" - the news was not good. They found cancer in one of my lymph nodes. So off we went down the path of chemotherapy, radiation and more chemotherapy for the next seven months.

Still Above Ground

<u>Timeline</u>

3.12.2018 to 10.4.2018
Tests, more tests, lots of tests

10.4.18	Bad news – cancer found in the lining of the uterus
10.22.18	The hysterectomy - just the beginning
10.29.18	Worse news – "the call" – cancer found in one lymph node Diagnosis: Stage 3 endometrial cancer
11.16.18	1st chemo treatment
11.22.18	The Thanksgiving un-feast
12.5.18	Hair gone
12.7.19	2nd chemo treatment
12.25.18	Bah humbug
12.28.18	3rd chemo treatment
1.24.19	1st day of radiation – it seemed so easy
3.4.19	28th day of radiation – bowel issues so bad it almost made chemo look easy
3.29.19	Hair beginning to grow back
4.12.19	4th chemo treatment
4.26.19	Bald again
5.2.19	5th chemo treatment
5.24.19	6th and final chemo – okay I'd rather go back to radiation day 28
5.31.19	70th birthday – too sick to celebrate

5.24.2019 (last chemo) to 5.24.2024 (five-year mark)
Tests, more tests, lots of tests

Table of Contents

Date	Title	Pg.
10.4.18	Setting the Stage	9
10.11.18	Getting Ready for Act 1	11
10.15.18	To Tell or Not to Tell	13
10.26.18	A-Frame	15
10.29.18	The Waiting Game	17
10.29.28	The Call	19
10.31.18	Optimism	21
11.1.18	The Flip Side	23
11.2.18	Window of Reality	25
11.6.18	Hair Today, Gone Tomorrow	27
11.7.18	CA 19-9	29
11.13.18	Perspective	33
11.14.18	The Haircut	37
11.16.18	Fear of the Unknown	39
11.17.18	Fear of the Known	41
11.19.18	Call 911: The Butter's Missing	43
11.20.18	You Look Good	45
11.21.18	Expectation	47
11.21.18	How Are You Doing?	49
11.22.18	Happy Thanksgiving	51
12.7.18	Thanks for the Memories	53
12.8.18	Post Pre-Cancer	55
12.11.18	Chemo Chair Haiku	59
12.12.18	No "Just" About It	61
12.14.18	I Have Cancer	63
12.15.18	The "What Ifs"	65

Still Above Ground

Date	Title		Pg.
12.28.18	I'm Fine	.....	67
12.29.18	Happy Holidays	.....	71
1.1.19	Happy 2019	.....	73
1.3.19	Pissed-O-Meter	.....	75
2.11.19	Did She Really Say That?	.....	79
2.19.19	Taking Care of Your Asshole	.....	83
3.4.19	I'm Too Young for This	.....	87
3.19.19	2019 Officially Blows	.....	91
4.3.19	Porcupine or Werewolf?	.....	93
4.9.19	Hello Bathroom My Old Friend	.....	96
4.13.19	Who Will I Be Today?	.....	99
4.15.19	Why?	.....	101
4.17.19	Low Point	.....	103
4.18.19	Turning the Corner	.....	105
4.19.19	Privilege	.....	107
4.20.19	The 2019 Unsung Hero Award	.....	109
4.24.19	Resilience	.....	111
4.26.19	A Shout Out	.....	115
5.3.19	Hair Loss Haiku	.....	117
5.8.19	I'm Just Not Myself Today	.....	119
5.28.19	Lower Point	.....	121
6.28.19	Bald Badge of Courage	.....	123
7.5.19	Chemo Brain	.....	125
10.4.19	Wrapping It Up	.....	127

Jeri Kroll

10.4.18
Setting the Stage
Thursday

I received the call this morning. Biopsy results from my hysteroscopy tested positive for cancer cells in the lining of my uterus aka endometrial cancer. Surgery would be scheduled as soon as possible. [*Little did I know what that call, those words, would mean for me.*]

After a few waves of emotion, mainly sadness and fear, I settled firmly into the denial phase of handling bad news. It must be an early diagnosis. It has to be. Surgery will take care of it. Just rip out the freaking uterus and ovaries and whatever else you find in there and what's left of me will be just fine. I haven't even been retired for a year. This can't be a repeat of what happened to Kelly just a couple of months ago ... or could it? Kelly was a 53-year-old former colleague who had just been promoted to CEO and died of lung cancer a mere 8 months after diagnosis.

When I asked the gynecologic oncologist, who called to inform me about my test results if he could tell me anything about the severity of the situation, he said they wouldn't know until after surgery when they would "stage" it. Honestly, the way he used the word "stage" as a verb threw me. I immediately pictured the stage of a play that was being set up for a live performance. What the heck's going on down there, I wondered. I pictured a group of tiny workmen with scaffolding and props entering my vagina squeezing their way up through my cervix into the

Still Above Ground

uterus followed by a troupe of actors and actresses eager to begin the first act. I sensed the performance would not be Tony Award worthy, but at least I hoped there would be plenty of comic relief.

Frankly, I'm hesitant to begin documenting my journey with cancer. After all, surely it will only be a one act play, a few unnoteworthy journal entries. But here I am and here I begin.

Jeri Kroll

10.11.18
Getting Ready for Act I
Thursday

Today my partner Jodi and I met with the surgeon who will be performing my hysterectomy. He was awesome. Thorough explanation of the type of cancer I have and how it normally behaves; thorough explanation of robotic surgery – what the procedure entails and the advantages; thorough explanation of the recuperation process and possible next steps. Plus, the real bonus - he had an excellent sense of humor. This means, of course, that he genuinely laughed at my jokes. Humor has emerged as my go-to approach to life in all its beauty and ugliness. For an appointment about cancer and surgery, there was a lot of laughter involved. If anyone is going to put sharp instruments into five incisions in my abdomen and suck my uterus out through my vagina, I want it to be someone with a good sense of humor!

Still Above Ground

"I do not wish my anger and pain and fear about cancer to fossilize into yet another silence, nor to rob me of whatever strength can lie at the core of the experience, openly acknowledged and examined ... imposed silence about any area of our lives is a tool for separation and powerlessness."

Audre Lorde
American writer and civil rights activist
The Cancer Journals
Breast cancer

Jeri Kroll

10.15.18
To Tell or Not to Tell – That is the Question
Monday

My surgery is one week from today and I haven't told many of my friends about the upcoming stage production that is about to occur. The dilemma is who to tell, who not to tell, who I would tell who would tell someone I didn't tell … it's quite complicated if you think about it. It's almost like planning a wedding except there are no gifts involved or seating plans to figure out.

I do have family and a few very close friends who know. They've also known about the multiple ultrasounds, MRIs, CAT scans, blood tests, endoscopies, hysteroscopy and for good measure colonoscopy leading up to the diagnosis. But there are a bunch of other friends and former colleagues who have no idea. For example, I had lunch last week with a woman from work, of whom I am quite fond, the day after I received "the call." I acted as if everything was perfectly normal – just back from a trip to Disney and The Wizarding World of Harry Potter at Universal with my partner, sister-in-law, younger nephew, older nephew and his fiancée - oh, yes, enjoying retirement. I did the same thing this morning when I chatted with our neighbor who was out walking her dog. "So, how's it going?" she asked as if she really wanted to know. "Great," I responded. "No complaints," I added enthusiastically.

Still Above Ground

The question is, when does a person cross into the I-really-should-let-them-know category? In hindsight I wished I had gone ahead and talked to the friend from work but probably not the neighbor – at least not now. Maybe I could just tone down my enthusiasm a bit about my supposedly carefree existence.

My task this afternoon is to make a list of people I know I'd regret not telling. After a lot of thought I've decided the determining question would be: if something like this were happening to them and they didn't bother to tell me, would I be upset? Would I think to myself, "Gee, I thought we were closer than that." It seems like a good approach.

Jeri Kroll

10.26.18
A-Frame
Friday

Surgery was four days ago – 7:30 a.m. sharp. My surgeon came in to talk with me that day around three o'clock in the afternoon after I'd been moved to a hospital room for a one-night stay. Surgery went well. Prognosis excellent. He added that I had brought an A frame to the table which made their job a whole lot easier. "Ok," I thought. "This is a sudden shift in imagery." Was the troupe of actors now building a chalet village in my vagina after my uterus, ovaries, a large fibroid tumor and a few lymph nodes were detached and extracted? I supposed there'd be room now, but it didn't seem like a particularly good time to start a construction project. Yet, images of snow peaked mountains and tiny skiers came to mind. "What the heck's going on down there now?" I asked out loud while I peered below at my abdomen. I was ready to be done with actors turned villagers. "I never liked A-frame construction," I warned whomever was listening, hoping no-one was. "I mean how do you hang your artwork on those steep sloping walls that go from roof top to ground floor with nary a perpendicular surface? And doesn't the heat just rise to the top of that stupid pointy roof?"

I know my doctor meant the frame imagery as a compliment but all I could think of were the many reasons A-frames, at least in my opinion (with no offense to anyone who owns one), are architecturally and aesthetically ridiculous structures.

"I've noticed that the people who are late are often so much jollier than the people who have to wait for them."
E.V. Lucas
English humorist and writer

"The more Susan waited the more the doorbell didn't ring. Or the phone."
Dirk Gently's Holistic Detective Agency

"Time is a funny and fickle thing. Sometimes there was never enough of it and other times it stretched out endlessly."
J. Lynn, author
Be with Me

Jeri Kroll

10.29.18
The Waiting Game
Monday Morning

It's been almost a week since surgery, and this may be the hardest part – waiting!

> Waiting for biopsy results
> Waiting for my body to move like it used to
> Waiting for people to stop treating me as if I'm incapacitated (even though I know they mean well).

Apparently many great and famous people have extolled the virtues of patience. Since I am neither great nor famous, I have evidently failed to incorporate this virtue into my character. Is it possible to become patient now on demand? Ironically, I cried, "I want patience and I want it NOW!"

So here I wait ... impatiently.

Still Above Ground

"It's strange how the worst day of your life often starts just like any other. You might even complain very quietly to yourself about its ordinariness. You might wish for something more interesting to happen ... and just when you think you can't bear the monotony any longer, something comes along that shatters your life to such degree you wish with every cell in your body that your day hadn't become so unordinary."

Joanna Cannon, British author
The Trouble with Goats and Sheep

10.29.18
The Call
Monday Afternoon

I just got "the call" this afternoon. Most of us have experienced at least one of these - the day everything changed. The surgeon just told me this was not going to be a one act play – not just surgery. Good thing I started a journal, I thought, but wondered if it had jinxed me. Honestly, I only took in a fraction of what the doctor was telling me. There was a lot of medical terminology with which I am completely unfamiliar. But more than that I was in a state of shock. As he said, "This isn't the news we were expecting." No shit!

What I did take in is that there were cancer cells in one of my lymph nodes which puts me on track for chemotherapy and radiation and also means this is beyond Stage 1. The other piece of information I understood was that there was something unusual about my cancer cells. They're sending my pathology report to the Cancer Review Board at Brigham and Women's Hospital in Boston who will discuss my case next week. Of course, I didn't know there was such a thing as a Cancer Review Board, but I must say it instilled some level of confidence in my medical care.

Here's my own staging:

The next best thing to not having cancer at all is having Stage 1 cancer.

Still Above Ground

The next best thing to having Stage 1 cancer is having a competent team of medical professionals to successfully navigate you through the higher stages.

The next best thing to having a competent team of medical professionals to successfully navigate you through the higher stages is feeling you've lived a full life without a bunch of regrets.

Of course, I'm trying not to let my mind go to that last "next best" thing, but I can't help it. Thoughts about how to put my affairs in order (not that I've ever had an affair) keep flitting into my mind. I wondered if anyone ever sent out RSVP invitations to their funeral ahead of time so you could see who would come.

In the meantime, I may need that crash course in patience as I wait for the Cancer Review Board to weigh in.

[*The report from Brigham and Women's was that my cancer cells were only slightly different – something about them being more mucous-y (my translation of some medical term) than usual, but I would receive the standard course of treatment. It turns out there was actually only one cancer cell. That's right - one fucking cell! The unfortunate reality is that one other cell might have gone somewhere else in my body and be multiplying as we speak – my pancreas, my esophagus, my brain?*]

10.31.18
Optimism
Wednesday

Most of my life people have labeled me as a "glass half empty" kind of person. I'm realizing this is just not true. I'm what I would call environmentally cautious. That's completely different from being a pessimist. For example, will I avoid standing on top of a hill in a thunderstorm or stay out of the water when there's been a shark attack? Of course! Do I assume the worst – that I will be struck by lightning or attacked by a shark. No!

Do I think I have one hell of a battle ahead of me? Yes! Do I think I should start planning my funeral even though I wonder who will come? No!

I find myself using words to describe the recent development in my situation as "not good" news. I don't say it's "bad" news. An optimistic person has "not good" news because with any luck not good news gets better. A pessimistic person has "bad" news because somehow bad news only gets worse.

Still Above Ground

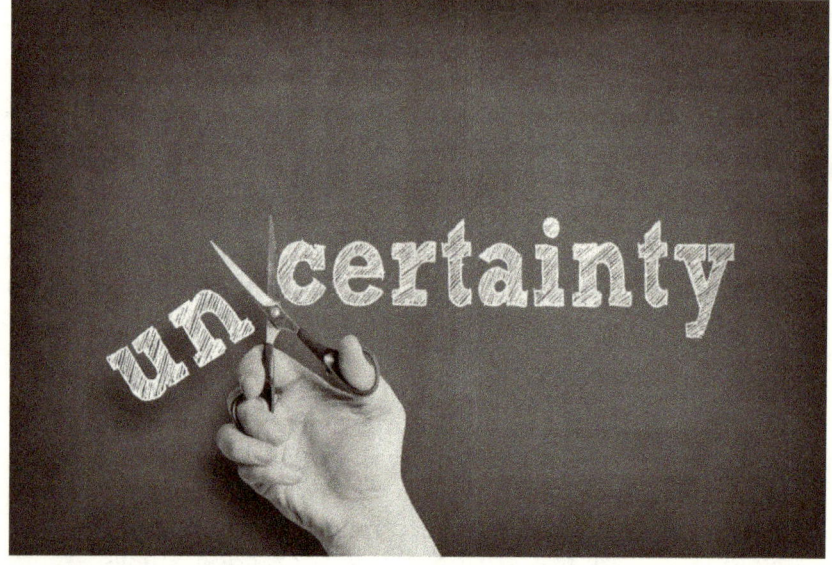

Jeri Kroll

11.1.18
The Flip Side
Thursday

Last night, out of the blue, a wave of overwhelming fear came over me. Fear of the future, fear of losing everything as I know it, fear that while I can put on a good front maybe I'm not that strong. What if I can't do this?

Still Above Ground

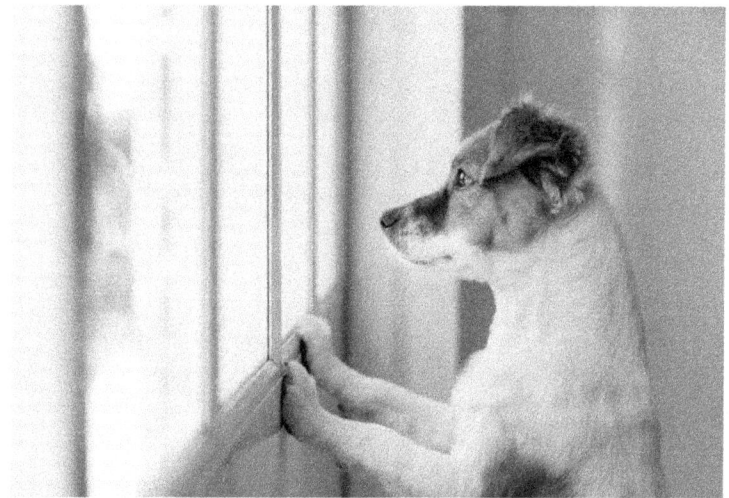

11.2.18
Window of Reality
Friday

This morning I feel quite peaceful. I'm warm. I'm safe. I have a hot cup of coffee and our dog snuggled up against me. I'm able to take in the love so many are sending my way which, for reasons I don't care to go into, is a miracle in and of itself. I was thrilled to get into the car this morning and drive for the first-time following surgery. So why was I overwhelmed by fear and anxiety last night and today I'm feeling so tranquil and calm?

I've been thinking about this all day and here's my conclusion:

It all has to do with which window of reality you're looking through. Many spiritual teachers, of course, have emphasized living in the now – focusing on the right here, right now window of reality. But, to me, living every day, every moment looking out that window is just not realistic. I have to think about the future. I have to make plans. I have to live in the real world. I have to look out of a larger window of reality where I can see more than what's right in front of me. Given my current situation looking out that larger window whether that's looking at next week, next month or, God willing, next year brings on a whole bunch of stressful considerations accompanied by a roller coaster of feelings.

Still Above Ground

So how do I decide which window I'll chose to look through at any given time, on any given day? Frankly, I have no idea. What I do know is that today, right here, right now I'm going downstairs, making a cup of tea, snuggling up with our dog and doing a crossword puzzle. No large window for me today!

11.6.18
Hair Today, Gone Tomorrow
Tuesday

Jodi and I met with the surgeon yesterday afternoon. We both left feeling reasonably hopeful and armed with a lot more information about my cancer and probable course of treatment. The bottom line, which I sort of already knew but was hoping was not the case, is that I'll be facing seven to eight months of chemotherapy and radiation.

And, "yes," the surgeon said, "you'll lose your hair." I suppose this is karma since for years I've poked fun at how much time and money humans spend on what's sprouting out of the top of their heads. I need to retract my statement that the number one fear, after the fear of public speaking, is the fear of a "bad hair" day. Clearly, the number one fear after the fear of public speaking is the fear of a "no hair" day!

I've been researching hats and scarfs for cancer patients. Apparently, it's a big industry with all the bells and whistles of marketing strategies aimed at making you feel that donning their stylish head coverings will render you indistinguishable from the non-cancer population. Who do they think they're fooling? The models wearing the hats or scarfs are all highly attractive younger women beaming with happiness as if it were their wedding day.

Still Above Ground

I will be purchasing some head wear, but I hold out no hope of looking anything at all like the models. [*I was so <u>not</u> wrong on this one!*]

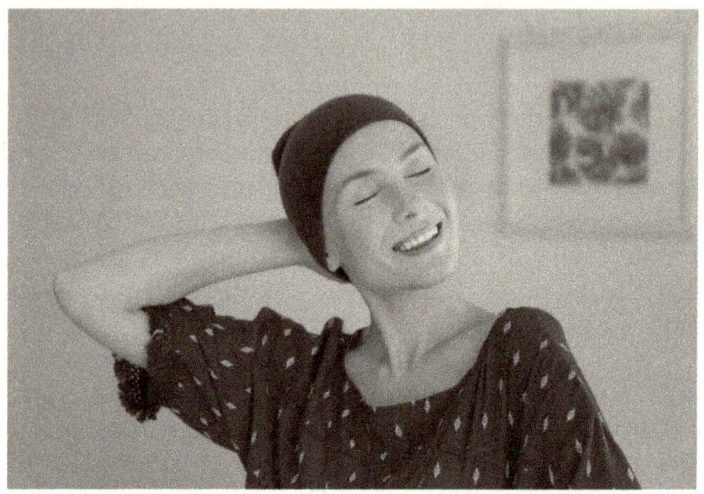

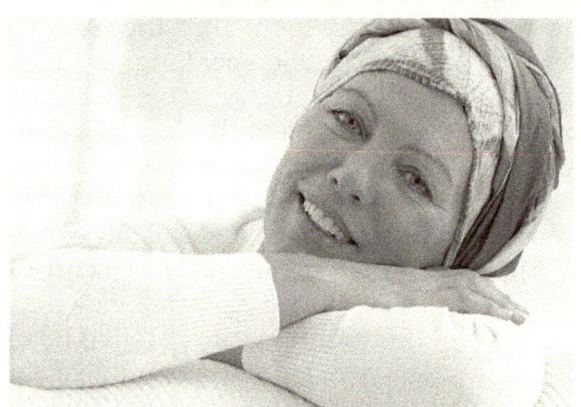

Jeri Kroll

11.7.18
CA 19-9
Wednesday

Last evening a message popped up on my iPad alerting me to a new lab result posted on my healthcare system's patient portal. I knew it was most likely the result of the blood work done following my appointment with the surgeon a couple of days ago. Frankly, I was both eager and petrified to check my chart. Here's why (and please excuse the "technical" nature of this entry).

Back in mid-April my lab work showed an elevated cancer antigen - specifically cancer antigen 19-9. Cancer antigens are proteins that exist on the surface of cancer cells which the cancer cells then shed. These can be measured in a person's blood stream. The presence of a whole bunch of these cells is obviously a red flag. The standard range for this particular antigen (CA 19-9) is ≤ 37. Mine was 132. So, since April my PCP has been chasing 19-9 trying to find out the source of the elevation. According to all the doctors to whom I was referred CA 19-9 is usually specific to the pancreas. The gastroenterologist I saw, however, was quite certain, after two endoscopies that although I do have a cyst on my pancreas, it was not a problem and not the source of CA 19-9. In one report he noted that other medical professionals "should look elsewhere for the source." Since no one could pinpoint that source my level was re-checked in July and it was still elevated at 130. In the back of my mind I decided we'd just have to ignore it since it seemed every crevasse of my body had been poked and prodded, tested and biopsied.

Then I started having very light, sporadic vaginal bleeding at which point my PCP immediately sent me back to the gynecologist. Although he took the bleeding very seriously, he was still certain it had nothing to do with CA 19-9. I was sent post-haste for a hysteroscopy. Biopsy results were positive for cancer cells in the lining of my uterus and I was promptly scheduled for surgery with a gynecologic oncologist. Following the operation as I was leaving my post-op appointment, the surgeon said to me almost as an afterthought, "Oh, yes, I'd be curious what happened to CA 19-9 now that you've had surgery. I'll send you down to the lab."

So that's the long winded, hopefully not too boring back story to the lab result I was expecting.

After receiving the email alert, I sat for a while – wanting to know and not wanting to know. If the number was still high that would mean that after all of this, I probably had cancer in some other part of my body. How would I handle that? Where would my sense of humor be then? I sat there awhile longer to weigh the odds that it is was good news vs. bad news. So many professionals were sure CA 19-9 usually had nothing to do with a women's reproductive organs. [*I hadn't yet learned that the word "usually" in the medical profession is kind of like the weather forecaster saying it would be a mixture of clouds and sun with the possibility of a snow shower depending on the speed and track of the cold front coming down from the north. "Usually" sometimes told me nothing. I write this with all due respect to the doctors and medical professionals I've seen in this process. They have usually been correct in their usually-s!]*

Finally, I gathered the courage to go upstairs to my computer. I logged on to my patient portal and clicked on the report labeled Cancer Antigen 19-9 dated 11/5/18. I looked at the result with one eye closed and one eye open. I figured that way if the news was bad, I could easily shut both eyes in a futile attempt to block out reality. Conversely, if the news appeared to be good, I could pop open both eyes to be sure I had seen the result correctly. To my astonishment both eyes confirmed that the number read 26. I was ecstatic! Of course, I ran upstairs at least four more times in the course of the evening to be sure I hadn't misread the number but every time I checked the number still read 26.

Although I still need chemotherapy and radiation, this is finally some good news!

Still Above Ground

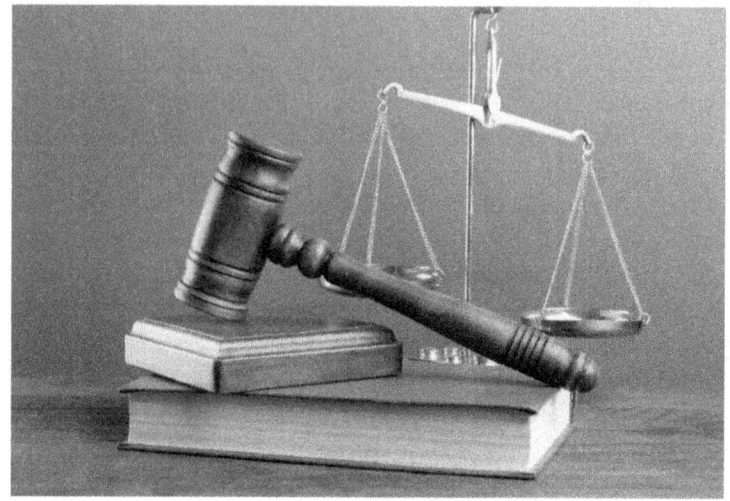

You have jury duty.

Jeri Kroll

11.13.18
Perspective
Tuesday

The sentence "you have jury duty" is right up there with the worst of all possible notifications. I decided to take my chances and not reschedule my date for jury duty even though it ended up being three days before I was scheduled for my first chemotherapy treatment. As everybody knows (at least in Massachusetts), you are often excused from service the day before when you call in to check on your status. In the event you do need to report, the day consists of an inordinate amount of waiting around, being shuffled from room to room and most often, when all is said and done, results in being excused from service. Unfortunately, I did need to report.

This morning about 90 grumbling humans arrived for jury duty at 8:00 a.m. at the Salem, Massachusetts District Court where we were checked in and assigned a number which was recorded in large print on a square card. I was juror #56. I promptly asked when I would have an opportunity to plead my case for dismissal. The clerk assured me there would be a time when prospective jurors would meet with the judge individually at which point, we could explain our specific circumstances. When everyone was checked in, all 90 of us were ushered into a large room where we viewed the movie about good citizenship and fulfilling our civic duty. Then we waited. Around 10:30 we were told that there were three cases up for trial – two in the District Court and one which was

Still Above Ground

actually in the Superior Court. The two District Court cases would be short and most likely not even go to trial. The Superior Court case would be longer and more complicated. Needless to say, I was hoping for one of the District Court cases but around 11:30 jurors #1 through #70 were moved to a different room for possible empanelment for the Superior Court case – assault and battery with a deadly weapon. We were told that testimony would probably run through Friday (my chemo day) with deliberation by the jury beginning on Monday. "Shit," I thought. "I could be royally screwed."

We were moved to yet another room where from 11:30 to around noon the 70 of us were asked a series of questions. If the answer was "yes", we were instructed to hold up our square number card. The majority of the questions had to do with how impartial we felt we could be given the nature of the case (domestic violence) and persons involved (black guy from Lynn, Massachusetts). Of course, since 8 a.m. I'd been hearing other members of the jury pool making up excuses to get out of serving and joking about how all you had to say was "Hang the bastard" and you'd be excused. Inwardly I had acknowledged my growing hostility toward my fellow potential jurors with their petty excuses. By the time half the jury pool held up their numbers indicating they could not be impartial, I was ready to explode. I had not held up my number because I felt I could be fair. (I like Lynn, Massachusetts. I used to live and work there. I voted to put up a Black Lives Matter banner at our church. Of course, I'm not a fan of domestic violence, but I'm liberal.) But what if, I thought, all the idiots who were just inconvenienced end up getting out of jury duty and by the time they get to me the judge says, "Sorry. I don't care if you have cancer and have to delay treatment. Everybody else is apparently a freaking racist."

After all the questions were asked and the numbers were recorded, we were taken in small groups to a different room beginning with juror #1 through juror #10. We learned that those 10 were then called individually to meet with the judge and either accepted or not accepted by the prosecuting and defense attorneys. I hoped that by the time they got to #50 to #60 a jury would have been empaneled but no such luck. When our small group of 10 was ushered into the smaller room, the lame excuses and stupid jokes resumed. When one woman lamented the fact that she had a European trip planned in two weeks and had soooo much to do, I couldn't stand it anymore! I decided they needed perspective! Totally uncharacteristically I announced that I had cancer and was scheduled to begin chemotherapy on Friday. One young woman actually gasped and blurted out, "Oh, my God, I'm so sorry." After that the room went silent.

Perhaps it wasn't fair of me. Who am I, after all, to determine what people "need?" [*Looking back this might have been the first of many "uncharacteristic" acts to come. Perhaps I should have realized then that this journey would result in many changes. It was definitely my first time using my brand new shiny "cancer card!"*]

When I was finally called before the judge around 3:30 in the afternoon, he graciously thanked me, excused me from service and wished me well.

Still Above Ground

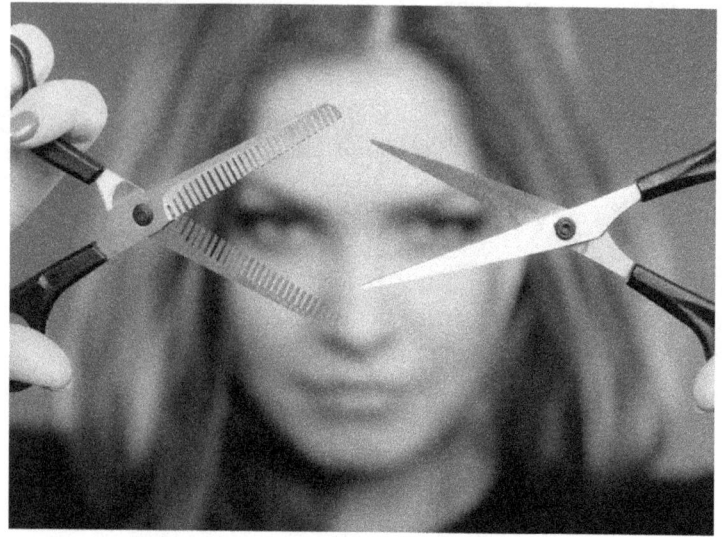

Jeri Kroll

11.14.18
The Haircut
Wednesday

I decided to get my hair cut really, really short today in preparation for the inevitable hair loss. Unexpectedly, everyone liked the new super short "do" and suggested this become my new style.

[*The haircut turned out to be a wise move. When my hair did start coming out right on schedule about three weeks after the first chemo treatment, it was still shocking. Short as they were, there were hairs everywhere. My partner complained that it was like living with a freaking cat. I love cats so that wasn't so much of a problem for me. The troubling part is that the hair loss is such an outwardly visible indicator of what chemo is doing to your body. It also immediately identifies you as someone who most likely has cancer. It's never been an identity you've ever wanted.*]

Still Above Ground

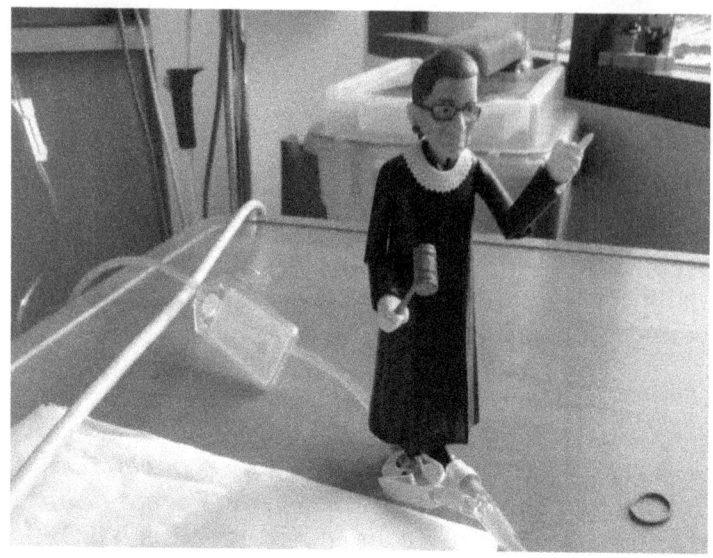

"I really concentrate on what's on my plate at the moment and do the very best I can."

Ruth Bader Ginsberg

Jeri Kroll

11.16.18
The Fear of the Unknown
Friday

Today is chemotherapy treatment #1. Apparently, this is a day-long event beginning with vitals, lab tests and a visit with the oncologist. This will be followed by the actual infusion of the chemo drugs (in my case carboplatin and taxol). This is scheduled for 3½ hours.

There are so many unknowns. Mainly, I've been trying to picture the physical layout of the infusion center. Would I be staring at 17 other patients in various stages of illness? Would some of them look skeletal like the stereotypical image of a person with cancer? Would it feel depressing or would I feel supported by the presence of others going down a similar path? Would they administer the chemicals through an IV or would I have a portal? Would any of it hurt? What should I wear? What should I take with me? And oh, yes, most importantly, what about lunch?

[*I'm not a superstitious person but I took an action figure of Ruth Bader Ginsburg with me to each chemotherapy treatment. RBG is quite popular at the time of this writing, at least among the more liberal folks! Aside from her political leanings, I took Ruth with me because she beat cancer twice – colorectal cancer in 1999 and pancreatic cancer in 2009. In December 2018 as I was finishing up my first three cycles of chemo, RBG also underwent surgery for early stage lung cancer.*]

Still Above Ground

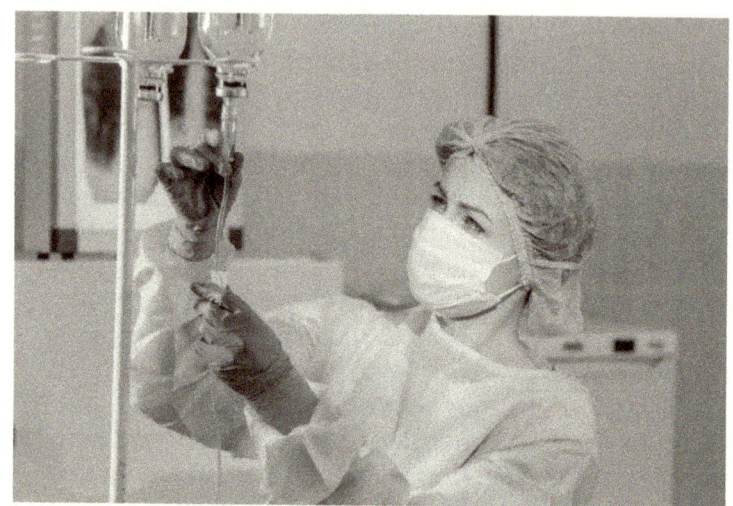

Jeri Kroll

11.17.18
The Fear of the Known
Saturday

Before I started chemotherapy, I told myself it was the fear of the unknown that would be the worst part. That has changed. The worst part of the next treatment will be the fear of what I know. It's not so much the actual infusion that's bad [*except when it takes an hour to find an acceptable vein*], it's the aftermath.

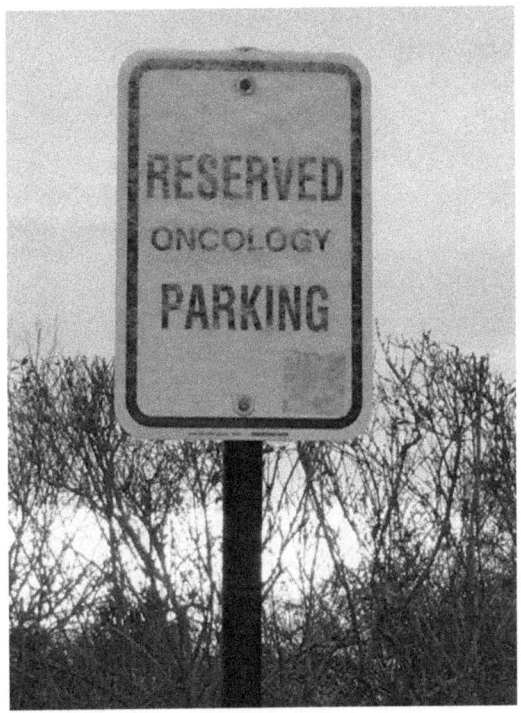

POP QUIZ #1

One of the greatest fears around having cancer is that:

    a. You will never be able to butter your toast again.
    b. Your OCD will get so bad you will need to take medication.
    c. You will be fined a large sum of money for abusing the 911 emergency response system.
    d. You will experience a loss of control and the inability to function as you have in the past.

Answer: _____

Jeri Kroll

11.19.18
Call 911 - The Butter's Missing
Monday

After two days of residing either in the bathroom or in bed, I emerged downstairs to the kitchen. I cannot deny that I am a control freak with perhaps a touch of OCD. When I go into the refrigerator, I expect to find items where I always put them. The upper left shelf, for example, houses certain dairy products – butter, cottage cheese, yogurt, sour cream. The top shelf on the door is host to all the condiments – ketchup, mayo, mustard, relishes. The rest of the fridge has designated areas for items similar in nature – beverages, veggies, salad dressings and so forth.

Today I managed to haul my sorry self downstairs to consume a piece of toast. When I reached into the upper left shelf to retrieve the butter, however, it was not there! I moved the sour cream to the right and the yogurt to the left hoping the butter was hiding somewhere behind its fellow dairy products. It was not! A more thorough search revealed that the butter had been placed on the bottom right shelf with, to my horror, the mustard.

I stood there taking in the scene as if a horrible accident had occurred. I calmed myself a bit with the thought of calling 911. What's the nature of your emergency? "Someone's been in the refrigerator and I found the butter and the mustard ***together*** on the bottom right shelf - please hurry."

Still Above Ground

In that moment I realized that loss of control has to be one of the hardest parts of having cancer. There are, of course, the big things over which you no longer have any choice or control, but equally important are the bazillion little things that result in your inability to be you.

And there was the terrifying question: if I lose control over the refrigerator, what's next?

Before eating my piece of buttered toast and returning to bed, I quickly reorganized the fridge so everything was back in its proper place.

Jeri Kroll

11.20.18
You Look Good
Tuesday

Today three days after the 1st chemo treatment when my partner told me at the dinner table that I looked good, I snapped! I felt like shit. "Why do people always want to tell sick people they look good?", I thought. "Do they think it makes you feel better? Does it make them feel better?" Right now, the last thing on my mind is how I look. I'm just trying not to projectile vomit onto someone else's dinner plate.

After my partner's unwelcome (and I would maintain inaccurate) observation, my response, said in a rather nasty tone, was something like, "Well, I'm glad for you that I look good, but I feel like crap." She snapped back, "Well, that was rude." I agreed and stormed away from the table throwing my plate in the sink and stomping upstairs to the bedroom.

Later, when reflecting on this unpleasant interchange, I realized I need to constantly keep in mind that cancer will also not be easy for the people around me. It's really not just about me.

While totally embracing that truth, I still wish that people would stop telling me how I look. I imagine having a T-shirt made that says, "Tell me how I look at your own risk." It would certainly curtail unwanted comments on my appearance. In fact, it would probably curtail any comments at all!

"The failure to think positively can weigh on a cancer patient like a second disease."
Barbara Ehrenreich
American author and political activist
Welcome to Cancerland
Breast cancer

"Cancer is not a straight line. It's up and down."
Elizabeth Edwards
American author and healthcare activist
Resilience: Reflections on the Burdens and Gifts of Facing Life's Adversities
Breast cancer

Jeri Kroll

11.21.18
Expectations
Wednesday – early morning

On the way to my radiology intake appointment this morning, I felt an intense sadness come over me and discovered tears streaming down my cheeks. "Oh shit," I mumbled. "So now I'm turning into a first-class bitch and an emotional basket case." Reluctantly, I decided I needed to "go with" the feeling and figure out what the heck was going on. [*I'm not a therapy graduate for nothing!*]

What I realized was that most of my life I've tried desperately to please other people – to live up to their expectations. For years I felt I fell short, that I was a disappointment. I continued to push harder and harder to prove myself. When I retired, a little over a year ago, I was in such a different place – feeling free from the need to demonstrate my worth over and over again. Upon entering this new world of cancer, the old nagging feelings of needing to prove myself, needing to fulfill other people's expectations, reared its ugly head. I was feeling pressure to be the strong Jeri, the brave Jeri, the "you-can-do-this" Jeri. I realized I couldn't go there. This journey can't be about other people's expectations. If ever there was a time to be solidly centered, it's now!

Still Above Ground

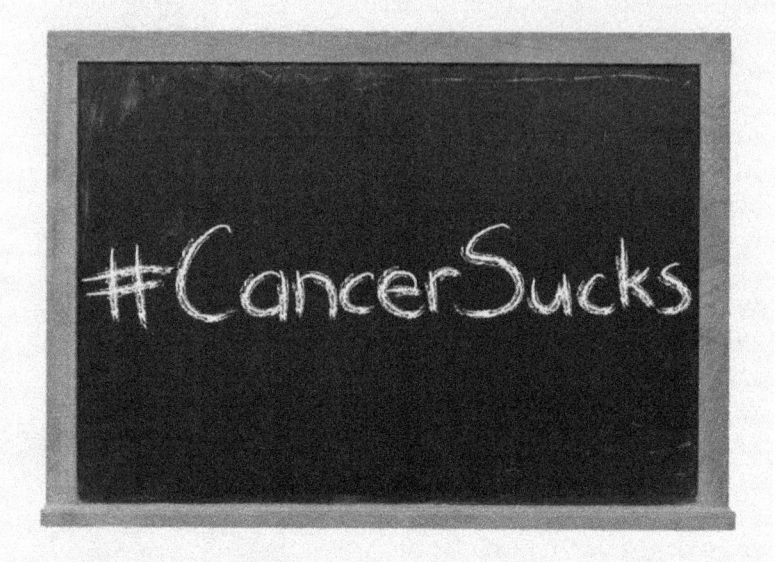

11.21.18
How Are You Doing with Your Diagnosis?
Wednesday – later morning

Today while attending my radiology intake appointment, both the nurse who saw me initially and the oncologist asked me how I was doing with my diagnosis. To be honest I wasn't sure why they were asking. Did they want to know if I understood my diagnosis or were they asking about my feelings? What did the word "doing" mean in this context? I decided in both instances it probably wasn't worth the mental effort to figure out why they were asking and just go with the truth. I responded by saying, "Well, it pretty much sucks." I wondered how other people might have answered. I can't imagine anyone saying, "I'm just thrilled with this turn of events in my life. It's the break I've been waiting for!" To be fair, I suppose part of good treatment would be to assess if a person needed some extra support. If someone said, "I'm devastated and can't go on," they might be referred to a social worker or some other helping professional.

I was relieved when both the nurse and the doctor seemed okay with my answer because it was the only response I could offer.

Still Above Ground

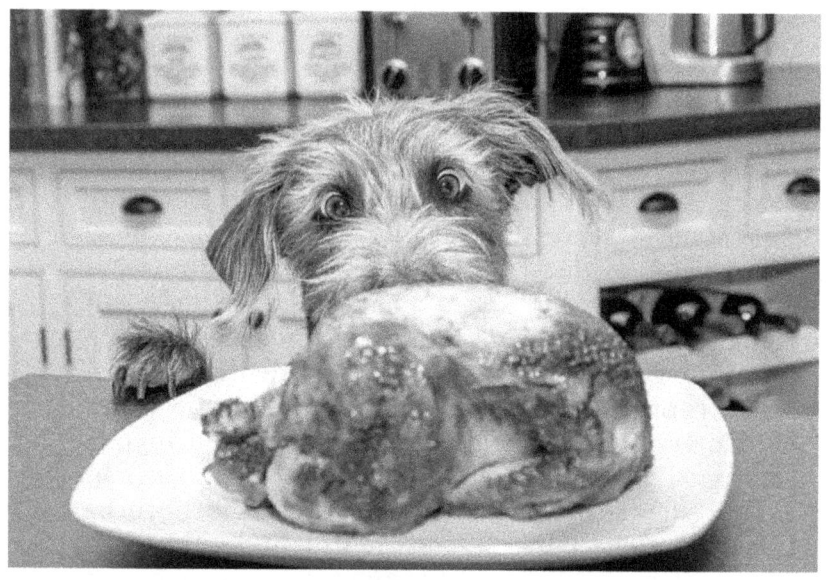

"Looks like an awesome Thanksgiving for me!"

Jeri Kroll

11.22.18
Happy Thanksgiving
Thursday

As I waited to be summoned for my radiology appointment yesterday, I was drawn to a man I had seen at the clinic before. Except for the fact that he had hair including a full, dark beard, he had cancer written all over him. Skinny to the point of skeletal, lethargic gait, dulled speech, struggling to carry a heavy plastic bag labeled Ensure. Hard to tell his age – maybe 50ish. He wore a dark blue beanie and was dressed in jeans and a plaid flannel shirt. Though lacking the requisite physique, he looked to me like a lumberjack. What I noticed most about him were his jet-black eyes. In a body that appeared half dead, his eyes were alive – observant and expressive.

As the would-be lumberjack entered the waiting room and sat down directly across from me, it quickly became obvious that he was well-known and well-liked by the staff. He was soon engaged in a lively conversation which turned to the subject of the upcoming Thanksgiving holiday. He asked one of the receptionists if she was having a big gathering to which she responded, "yes," and went on in great detail about the number of people coming and the events of the day. At the end of her monologue my fellow cancer patient mumbled wistfully, "Yeah, right, me too ... and they'll all be asking, 'Oh, how're you doin'?'" His voice mimicked how they would sound – polite, superficial – not really looking for or wanting an answer. Then, not in a mean way, but

Still Above Ground

in a way that said, "I've resigned myself to fit into your social gathering," he sighed, "Yeah, right."

At that point I couldn't help but smile. I understood completely. As I looked up at him our eyes locked. Those jet-black eyes smiled back at me and he nodded. No words necessary. Happy Thanksgiving.

Jeri Kroll

12.7.18
Thanks for the Memories
Friday

When I was about 12 years old my parents sent me for swimming lessons at the community pool. For some reason, trapped in some suppressed memory, I was petrified of the water. Though I obediently put on a swimsuit, when the moment of departure came, I decided I was NOT going for swimming lessons. And so it was that my older brother and his buddy were tasked with delivering me poolside. As they tried to get me into the car and subsequently extract me from the vehicle to escort me down the hill to the pool, my arms, legs, fingers and toes wrapped themselves around any available stationary object – a fence post, the car door, a light pole, a tree. There was a lot of finger peeling involved. Upon eventually arriving at the pool, my memory is that the swim instructor told the boys to simply throw me in the deep end. I hope my memory is a bit off on that detail, but it wouldn't surprise me since we definitely lived in a "sink or swim" kind of world back then.

Going for the second chemo treatment felt exactly like being escorted to the pool – desperately wanting to cling to anything to prevent the inevitable. I wondered what would happen if I actually clung on to one of the pillars in the car port at the entrance to the oncology center. It was certainly an amusing image. I wondered - would two teenage boys suddenly appear to peel me off the pillar and throw me into infusion chair #11?

Still Above Ground

[*Unfortunately, I lacked the courage to actually go to the Cancer Center and pose with my body wrapped around the pillars.*]

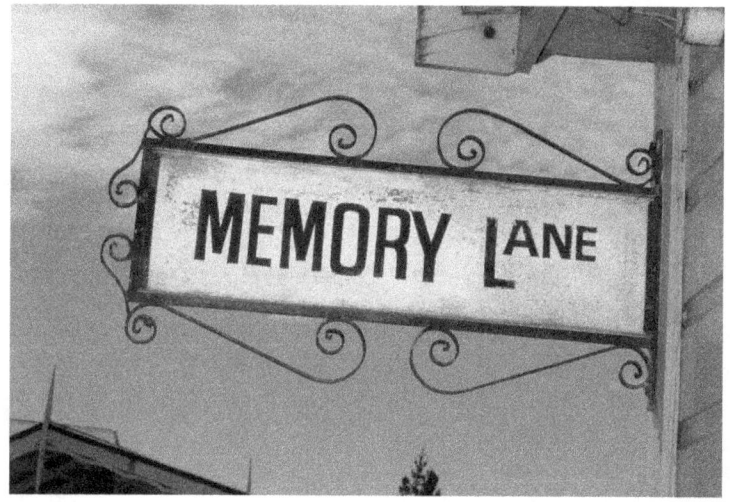

Jeri Kroll

12.8.18
Post Pre-Cancer
Saturday

Oddly, it hadn't occurred to me until today to ask my oncologist one big obvious question – when all of this is over – the chemotherapy, the radiation treatments, more chemotherapy – when it's all done, how will I know if it's been successful? In other words, when can I declare myself a survivor?

The doctor was right when she told me I wouldn't like the answer. "It's a waiting game," she said. The God damned waiting thing again, I lamented. The bottom line is that if no more nasty cancer cells crop up in the next five years then the treatment is considered effective. Not "liking" the answer was an understatement! Five years? Five years of not knowing. Really? I'll be 75 years old at that point. For God sake, by then I could be dead from some other dreadful disease.

I wondered when other people with cancer called themselves survivors. There certainly seem to be a lot of folks running around using the term. Do I have to wait five years for a "post-cancer" diagnosis to call myself a survivor?

I did what I always do in these situations, I made a beeline to the internet and typed in the search box "when do people with cancer call themselves survivors". Sure enough the first hit was an article called "Am I a Cancer Survivor?" by Kathy Latour.* That and numerous other articles pointed me to an interesting organization called the National Coalition

Still Above Ground

for Cancer Survivorship which was founded in 1986. One main goal of the coalition was to change the language we use when referring to people with cancer from "victim" to "survivor." Thankfully, their campaign has been hugely successful as it has helped to shift the way others see and treat those of us with cancer and even more importantly how we see and treat ourselves. Nobody wants to be a victim.

Although my detour into the National Coalition for Cancer Survivorship's website was interesting and informative, it still did not address my question about the when of it – when can I call myself a survivor? I returned to Ms. Latour's article in which she confirms that this confusion is common. She maintains, "it starts the day you hear the word 'cancer'." Apparently not all survivors are satisfied with that answer because they don't like being lumped together with all other survivors and want some differentiation. Some professionals have identified and assigned labels for four types or stages of survivorship. Maybe I'll feel differently later, but right now this all seems rather crazy.

I agree with Kathy (she doesn't know it but we're on a first name basis now) when she says, "Overall, it just makes sense to live life to the fullest no matter what one wants to call us, because cancer can't stop that no matter how hard it tries." Yay, Kathy!

I also looked up the word "survivor" in several reputable dictionaries. Uniformly they define "survivor" as "a person who is able to continue living their life successfully despite experiences of difficulty." In other words, a survivor is someone who is surviving

- present tense, not someone who survived – past tense.

So, it seems I have my answer. By all accounts I can declare myself a survivor now – no matter what type or stage I am. I now think of my life as pre-cancer and post pre-cancer – just those two phases. There's really no need to wait impatiently for five years to pass so I can declare a post-cancer phase.

*Published April 19, 2017 in "Cure Today". Ms. Latour (Kathy) is a breast cancer survivor, author of the "Breast Cancer Companion" and co-founder of CURE Magazine.

Still Above Ground

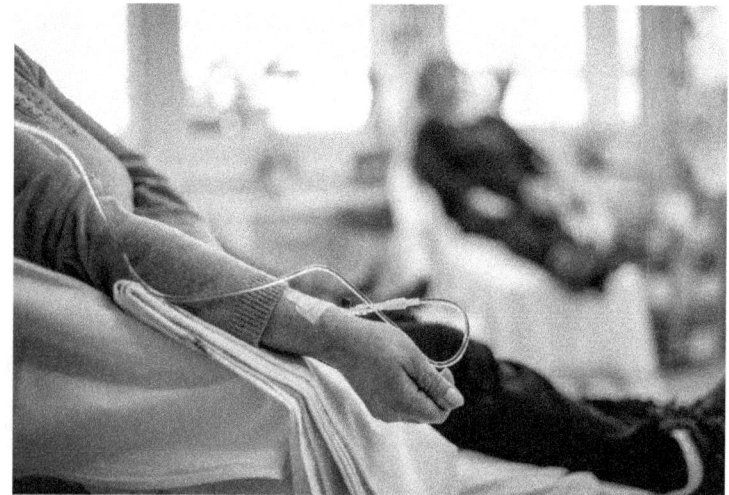

Jeri Kroll

12.11.18
Chemo Chair Haiku
Tuesday

Comfy looks deceive
Soft, reclining chair of pain
Poison stands ready

Still Above Ground

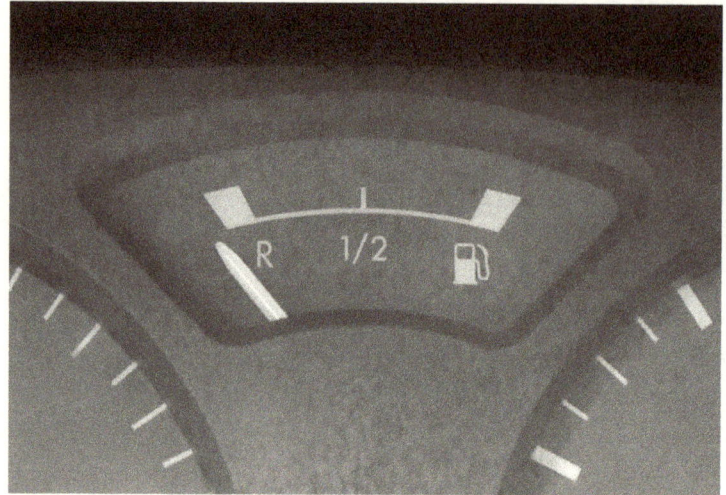

Running on Empty

Jeri Kroll

12.12.18
No "Just" About It
Wednesday

While the first couple of days after Chemo #2 were better than I expected, I lapsed into a state of absolute exhaustion. I had experienced this to some extent before except for a shorter period of time. After Chemo #1 when I told people I was feeling fatigued, I'd been met with various reactions including, "Well, at least you're not sick" or "That's good, you can just sleep if you need to." I understand those responses. They would have been mine a month ago. I had no clue, I mean no clue, what exhaustion could mean. My frame of reference was pulling an all-nighter or two in college when you were getting ready for finals or suffering from jet lag after a long flight across multiple time zones. Like it or not (mainly not), my perspective, my frame of reference, has totally and permanently changed.

The best way I have to describe the level of exhaustion I'm experiencing is that if I fell crossing a street and suddenly a tractor trailer was barreling down the road toward me, I'm not sure I would have the energy to move. Seriously. It's not that I wouldn't want to move or that I've developed some sort of grotesque death wish, but I'm literally not sure that I could. The insidious part of the whole thing is that as much as you sleep, you wake up in the same state – no more rested, no less exhausted. It's like a battery that won't recharge no matter how long you leave it plugged in.

Still Above Ground

When I mustered enough energy to sit up for a while this afternoon, I looked on the internet to see what others had to say about fatigue and cancer. It was validating to find that this level of exhaustion is very common. The Cleveland Clinic website states fatigue is "the most common side-effect" and describes it as "paralyzing." Confirming my battery analogy, they go on to say, "It comes on suddenly, does not result from activity or exertion and *is not relieved by rest or sleep.*" And, can you believe it, even more affirmation came from the American Cancer Society? "The fatigue that comes with cancer, cancer related fatigue (CRF), is *not the tired feeling people remember before they had cancer.* People describe feeling weak, listless, drained or 'washed out'." CRF? Really?

I'm sure if I started saying I have CRF everyone would think I was just using some new three letter excuse to go back to bed. Personally, I'm pretty sure I won't take up using the term, but I realize there *is* a word I need to stop using – the word "just". When asked how I'm doing I often respond, "I'm just tired" or "I'm just feeling exhausted." But there's no "just" about it. I'm not "just" exhausted. I'm exhausted. Eliminating the word "just" probably won't do a thing to enhance other people's understanding but I think I'll feel a tad bit better about myself if I can make this change. I'm not sure why I'll feel better, but right now if I feel a tad bit better about anything, for any reason, at any time – I'll take it!

Jeri Kroll

12.14.18
I Have Cancer
Friday

Yesterday I had lunch with a former colleague and, as one might expect, the topic of conversation turned to the trials and tribulations of the workplace. It was about the usual stuff that seems to occur in all places of employment – difficult personalities, communication issues, endless, senseless meetings, hidden agendas, elephants in rooms. At one point, since I'm retired and no longer need to deal with this stuff, I blurted out, "Geez, it makes me glad I have cancer." The moment it came out of my mouth, of course, I was appalled. Talk about invalidating another person's experience. As if that wasn't bad enough, I had played the cancer card when I didn't even mean to. My friend responded by saying that, of course, she didn't have it that bad. I tried to make some lame excuse for why I made the statement in the first place. I departed the restaurant wondering if the relationship would be permanently damaged. [*Miraculously, it was not.*]

On the drive home I confirmed with myself that I was indeed an asshole. [*Honestly, I knew this way before cancer!*] The question that arose for me, however, was whether or not cancer was becoming my world. Is this the beginning of a new identity? Will my every waking moment be filled with thoughts about cancer – the cure for cancer, cancer research, cancer support groups, cancer walks? Will I become oblivious to the hundreds of other diseases and life altering situations that people face? Will it only be about me and my struggle?

Still Above Ground

I hope not. I'm sure I will get involved in some cancer related activities and one day publish my journal, but I hope cancer doesn't take up any more of my life than it already has.

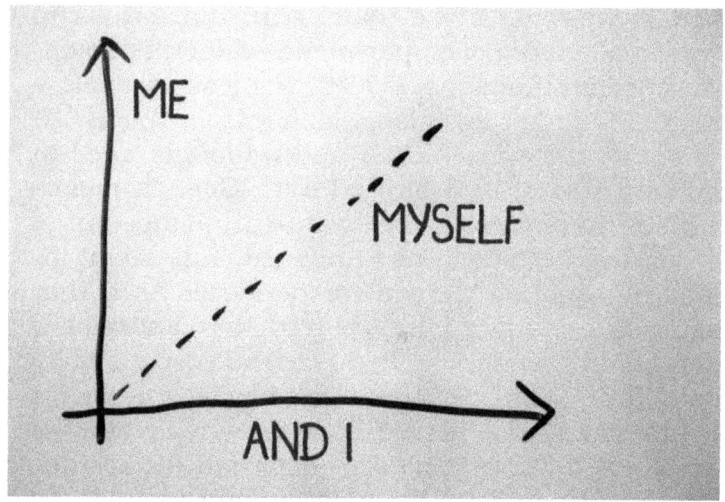

Jeri Kroll

12.15.18
The "What-Ifs"
Saturday

It's been a little over two months since my diagnosis and, so far, I've remained quite positive. In the past couple of days, however, I've felt a bit of doubt creeping in. What if the chemo and radiation treatments aren't effective? What if that one cell was not just one but many? What if I have cancer multiplying in my body as we speak? What if the diagnosis was not in fact early but late? What if I'm fooling myself into thinking this will all have a happy ending and by summer I'll be traveling down the path toward wellness?

Before surgery the oncologist was very certain that a hysterectomy would be all that I needed. No reason to think otherwise. Right after surgery the same thing – everything looked good, nothing of concern. One week later a different story – oh wait, a slight problem with a lymph node. What if there's another "oh, wait" about to be dropped in my lap?

I'm realizing that these "what-ifs" could easily have a paralyzing effect on me even though on many levels they're natural and reasonable. It's just that I'd rather not feel paralyzed right now in addition to everything else.

What occurs to me is that not all "what-ifs" are created equal. Some "what ifs" are solidly based in reality and there's something you can do about them proactively or preventatively. Other "what ifs" are just exacerbated fears of the unknown and

Still Above Ground

there's really nothing you can do. I think my "what-ifs" right now are more of the second type. The fear that treatment won't be successful is just that – a fear of the unknown.

My hope is that although I know this fear will rear its ugly head from time to time, it will not paralyze me or prevent me from enjoying my life. Right now, it seems like a lofty goal!

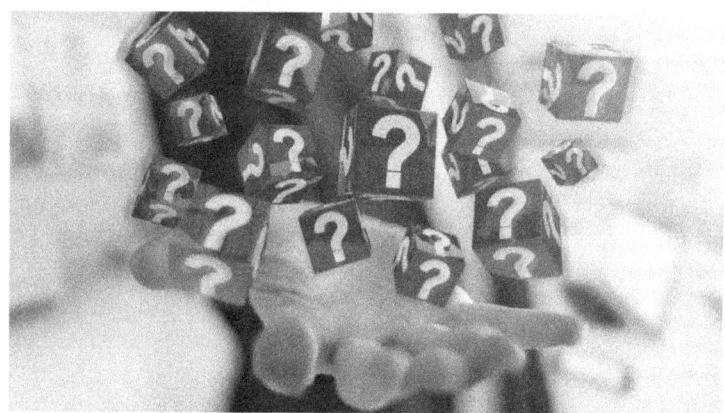

Jeri Kroll

12.28.18
I'm Fine
Friday

As I entered the Cancer Center this morning for Chemo Treatment #3, five hospital staff – two receptionists, two nurses and one phlebotomist, greeted me with a cursory, "Hi, how are you?" Do they really want an answer? They do know they work with cancer patients, don't they?

Twice I acquiesced to the social norm and said with little to no affect, "I'm fine." Once I pretended I didn't hear the question and didn't answer. It didn't seem to matter. Once I said, "I'm really not sure" which elicited a puzzled look. On the fifth encounter, I replied, "Still above ground" which is now my favorite phrase, but on this particular morning it was received without any appreciation of its implicit humor.

I've gone on rants about this before – pre-cancer – because it seems to me most often people aren't actually asking you how you are and aren't really looking for an answer. It's just a redundant way of saying "hi". In my current world, despite the early morning interactions with the two receptionists, two nurses and one phlebotomist, I'm experiencing a different reality. *Sometimes when a person asks you how you are, he or she actually wants to know!*

I have two oncologists – a medical oncologist and a radiation oncologist. When one of these doctors asks me how I am, she really wants to know, and I truly believe it's not just because it's her job. More importantly when people in my personal support network ask me how I am, they too are genuinely asking.

Early on in this journey when one of the doctors asked me how I was doing, I answered with my standard response - "I'm fine". She immediately looked me straight in the eye and said, "No, really tell me how you are." I'm not sure if it was the eye contact or the sincerity in her voice, but I was deeply touched. I left that appointment with a lump in my throat and the beginning of a bad headache, like what happens when you're at the movies and somebody's dog dies and you have to fight like hell to avoid bawling in public.

At a subsequent appointment, I was about to proceed with the "I'm-fine" routine but I stopped myself. Instead I described my physical being which included a report on my level of fatigue, a delightfully detailed description of my bowel movements and so forth. "Good", I thought, "You're making progress." The doctor, however, pressed even further by asking, "And, how are *you*?" Really, how am *I* as in how is the *me* of me? Come on, it's bad enough you have cancer. Your oncologist shouldn't make you feel all blubbery, so you leave her office with a knot in your throat and a migraine brewing.

Of course, there will still be the folks who are merely following the social norm when they ask how you are. Because of my enlightening post pre-cancer experiences, I'm going to try to start answering people when they ask. Some, I'm sure, will be sorry they inquired. I may say "still above ground" or I may say "I feel like shit" or I may say "I'm having an exceptionally wonderful day" but for the life of me, I hope I will stop saying, "I'm fine."

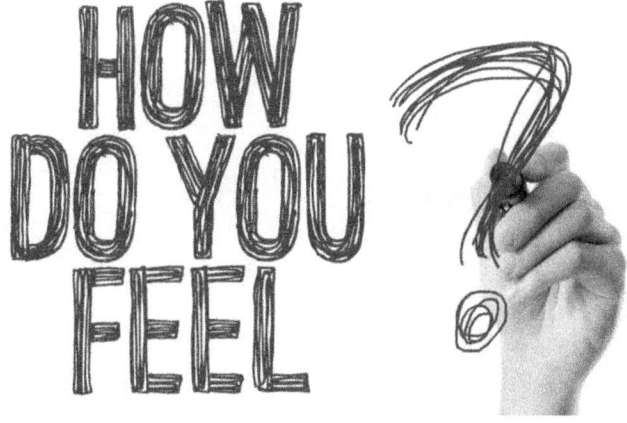

Still Above Ground

POP QUIZ #2

These are some of the cards I received during the holidays. Which was my favorite?

A.

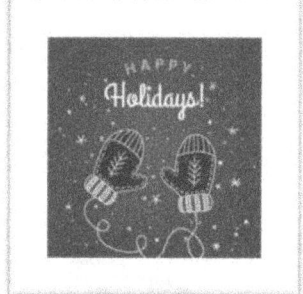

B.

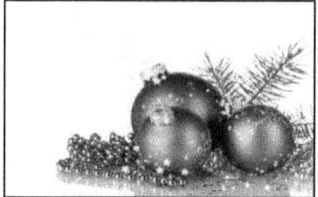

MERRY CHRISTMAS

C.

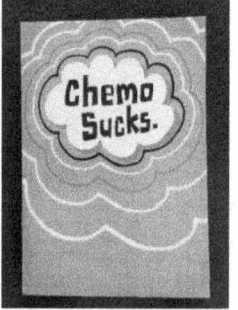

ANSWER: _____

Jeri Kroll

12.29.18
Happy Holidays
Saturday

Today my body is completely lethargic and all food choices sound disgusting. But as I lay in a heap upon my bed with our trusty dog at my side, my thoughts are whirling about. They landed on the fact that there really should be Christmas carols and movies written specifically for cancer patients who find themselves in the throes of chemotherapy in this oh so wonderful time of the year. Titles of more appropriate carols might include:

> O Chemo All Ye Faithful
> Deck the Halls with "Bowels" of Folly
> Up on the Rooftop Santa Barfs
> It's Beginning to Look a Lot Like Nausea
> Oh, There's No Place Like My Bathroom for the Holidays

Some movie titles might include:

> Home Alone – For Good Reason
> Fatigue Actually
> Nausea on 34th Street
> How Chemo Stole Christmas
> While You Were Sleeping (title perfect; significant plot change)

I decided to change the words to a few Christmas carols so that I, too, could sing merrily and embrace the holiday spirit.

Still Above Ground

Here's one example:

<u>Chemo Bell Rock</u>
(Sung to the tune of Jingle Bell Rock)

Chemo bell, chemo bell, chemo bell rock
Chemo bells swing on the oncology wing
Flowing then dripping through IVs with drugs
Now the chemo rock has begun.

Chemo bell, chemo bell, chemo bell rock
Chemo bells chime in chemo bell time
Flowing then dripping in Cancer Bell Square
In the clinic there.

What a bad time yet it's the "right" time
To live through this nightmare
Chemo bell time is a swell time
To go rocking in a chemo chair.

Giddy-up chemo nurse, pick up your feet
Chemo around the clock
Mix and a-mingle to the chemo bell beat
That's the chemo bell
That's the chemo bell
That's the chemo bell rock.

1.1.19
Happy 2019
Tuesday

I'm not a big Facebook user, but I'm avoiding it altogether today. Too many optimistic assholes embracing their "best year EVER!" Well, good luck and #@$#@ you!

Still Above Ground

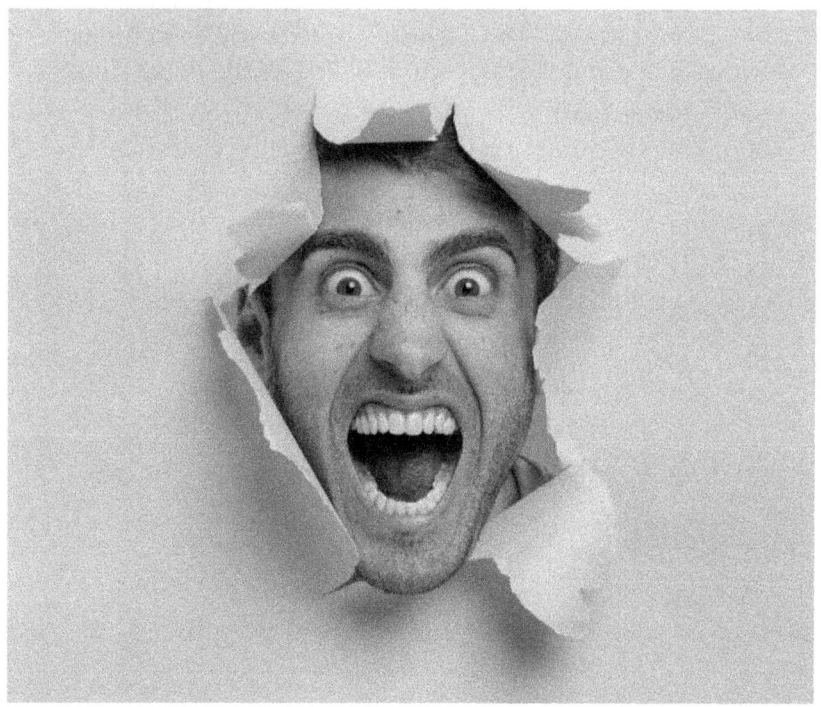

Jeri Kroll

1.3.19
Pissed-O-Meter
Thursday

It's Day #6 after chemo treatment #3. I woke up feeling grouchy and out of sorts. This morning when someone commented that at the six-day mark I "should be feeling better," my irritability level shot through the roof. I decided I needed to create my own irritability rating scale which I would call the Pissed-O-Meter.

There are, of course, already an existing number of rating scales that gauge a person's level of anger. These tools have been developed by psychologists and other mental health professionals primarily, from what I can tell, to create an anger management plan. The goal is to assess the types of situations that evoke the anger response and strategize about how to handle them. The goal of my Pissed-O-Meter would be primarily to embrace and accept myself at whatever level I am on any given day, for any given reason, in any given circumstances. Once identifying and accepting my irritability level, the steps toward self-management could be flushed out – or not.

The statements on the Pissed-O-Meter scale reflect how I would like to (but don't) verbalize my feelings of irritability toward other people. On a scale of 1 – 10 they are:

1. Leave me alone.
2. Don't talk to me.

3. There are no stupid questions, except yours. Yours are really stupid.
4. You are so wrong, about so many things, on so many levels.
5. Mind your own fucking business.
6. Don't tell me how I look. How many times do I have to tell you, I don't care how I look to you? It has no bearing on how I am or how I feel or how I'm actually doing.
7. Please remove yourself from my presence or I may need to poke an eye out – preferably yours.
8. I need to scream now. Perhaps it will drown out the voices – yours and the ones in my head.
9. If you tell me a story about your Aunt Betty's cancer, I will harm you. I know you mean well but understand this – I am not Aunt Betty. No other cancer patient is Aunt Betty. None of us ever liked Aunt Betty and there's a good chance the only thing we have in common with Aunt Betty is that we're all assholes.
10. Call 911 and tell them it's urgent that I be locked up before it's too late.

I haven't yet talked with many other people who have or have had cancer, but I suspect irritability is a major "problem" for a lot of us. One precipitating event, like someone saying you should be feeling better, can leave you (or me at least) feeling hostile and asocial for way longer and way more intensely than it normally would. At heart, you actually like people – well, most of them – well, a subset of them – well, sometimes a few of them. Oh, screw it – I'm still at a nine just remembering the "should be feeling better" incident. Best thing for me right now would be to take a long walk - alone.

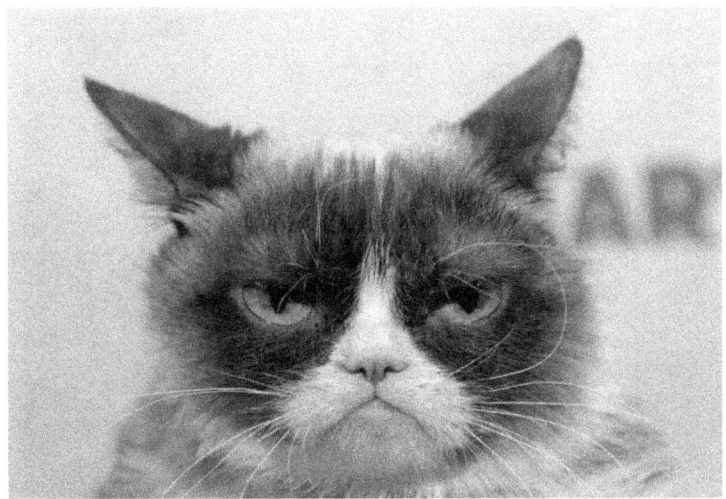

Still Above Ground

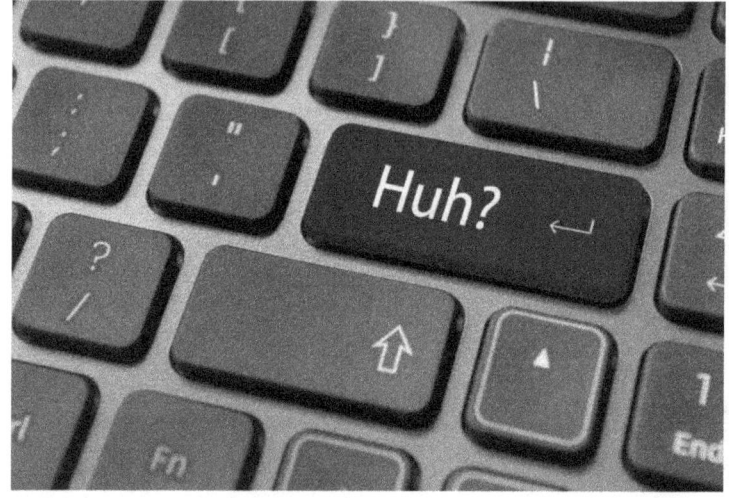

Jeri Kroll

2.11.19
Did She Really Say That?
Monday

Last week the Ipswich Council on Aging (COA) hosted a presentation by the local YMCA about two programs the Y offers for people with cancer and their families – Corner Stone and Live Strong. Both these programs include a free one-year membership to the Y as well as other benefits such as special exercise classes, educational presentations and support groups. Before cancer I had started to swim twice a week at the Y through the Council on Aging for a small daily fee without needing to pony up the money for a full membership. I was excited to learn about these two programs.

As I waited at the Senior Center for the informational session to begin, I was surprised to count 18 other older women gathered. I assumed the group would be a bit more diverse. It quickly became evident that the group consisted of regulars at the COA who heard that some sort of presentation was happening and, perhaps having nothing better to do, meandered over to see what it was about.

When the nice representative from the Y began her talk by explaining that the programs she was presenting were specific to individuals with cancer, she was interrupted mid-sentence by the woman sitting next to me who said angrily, "What we want to know is why there is no discount for seniors." Seventeen other seniors muttered sounds of agreement.

Still Above Ground

The nice young representative from the Y explained that a senior discount wasn't available right now but was certainly something that should be considered in the future. As she tried to return to her talk about the programs for individuals with cancer, the same woman sitting next to me interrupted again by demanding, "I thought this was about programs that benefit seniors." Yes, again seventeen other seniors muttered their expressions of agreement.

The nice young, patient representative from the Y explained again that she was there to talk about programs specific to individuals with cancer. She actually managed to briefly explain some of the basics of the two programs. Realizing that no one else gave a shit about these benefits, I quickly thought about what information I needed and raised my hand. "I have cancer," I explained. "What I want to know is when can I sign up? I'm in active treatment now so I'm afraid I won't have the energy to take full advantage of either program. Can I sign up after I'm finished with chemotherapy?" The answer was that I could wait until I completed treatment and I'd still be eligible for the full year of membership. "Awesome," I thought.

When the nice young, patient, persistent representative from the Y tried to continue with her presentation, the same woman sitting next to me again interrupted mid-sentence. She shot me a sideways glance and announced in a huff, "Well, I don't want to have cancer to get some kind of a break." Third verse same as the first - seventeen other seniors muttering sounds of assent.

I blinked my eyes several times as my mouth opened to voice a response. All I could manage to

Jeri Kroll

snarl, as I glared back at her was. "No, you don't want to have cancer." My eyes blinked a few more times, I crossed my arms and disappeared into my private chemo brain. As soon as the presentation was over, I fled to my car and sped home.

Later when I thought about what happened, I questioned myself several times. "Did she really say that? Can people really be that insensitive and self-absorbed?" Every time the answer was the same. "Yes, she did say that and, yes, people can be that insensitive and self-absorbed."

[*I did sign up for the Corner Stone program which is awesome. I hope the eighteen senior assholes – the one big verbal asshole and the seventeen little assenting ones - get their senior discount. Maybe about the time my unfair "cancer membership" ends, I can take advantage of the senior discount. Of course, there will be other insensitive, self-absorbed folks out there who will mutter angrily, "I don't want to have to be old to get some kind of a break."*]

POP QUIZ #3

True or False

(T) or (F)
circle one

In preparation for meeting with your oncologist you should practice using professional, anatomically correct terminology like "rectum" and "anus" in your everyday language.

Jeri Kroll

2.19.19
Taking Care of Your Asshole
Wednesday

While I was in the shower this morning preparing to go to radiation treatment #19 out of 28 –(not that I'm counting), I thought about the conversation I did *not* have with my oncologist yesterday. The fact is when referring to my body parts I speak in Plain English. My doctor always refers to those parts or those bodily functions using anatomically correct terminology. For example, she asks me about urination and bowel movements not about pee and poop. Given my ongoing difficulty with diarrhea, I knew the subject of rectal care should be discussed. The problem was at the time the only word that came to mind in referring to this part of my anatomy was "asshole" not "rectum" or "anus." I supposed it would be inappropriate for my doctor, who also happens to be the head of the Radiology Department, to turn to me and ask, "So, how's your asshole?". I felt I needed to maintain her standard of civility. And, thus, I was rendered speechless.

If only the words "rectum" or "anus" were a part of my everyday vocabulary, I thought. I decided I needed practice. When I played it out in my head, however, I encountered some difficulty. For example, when another driver cuts you off in traffic you just can't shout out "you rectum." Even the more refined among us would utter a hearty "you asshole." After considering many possible combinations of words that would assist me in modifying my vocabulary, the phrase I like best is " flaming anus." It has sort of a poetic ring to it. It uses an F word without using *the* F word and it uses the word anus instead of asshole. I can definitely see myself using the phrase ... and just for amusement, I have!

Because I was not successful in discussing rectal care with my doctor, I reviewed the informational materials provided to me by the oncology team. As expected, the words used to provide the necessary information were very professional. In the manual, "Radiation and You: Support for People with Cancer" prepared by the National Cancer Institute, I quickly found the section on "Taking Care of Your Rectal Area" under "Radiation Side Effects: Diarrhea." It reads:

"Instead of toilet paper, use a baby wipe or squirt water from a spray bottle to clean yourself after bowel movements. Also, ask your nurse about taking sitz a bath, which is a warm-water bath taken in a sitting position that covers only the hips and buttocks. Be sure to tell your doctor or nurse if your rectal area gets sore."

I thought the National Cancer Institute would welcome my services in translating their manual into a more user-friendly version for those of us who are ill-equipped to use proper medical terms. Here is a sample of the above translated into PE (Plain English):

"Toilet paper is not your friend. Go to your local discount store and buy a shit load of baby wipes and a squirt bottle. After you take a dump, squirt your asshole with water or use a baby wipe or two to clean the area. Also, ask your nurse about taking a sitz bath. Although they sound similar, do not confuse

Jeri Kroll

"sitz" with "shits". "Sitz" is a fancy word for plopping your sorry ass in warm water. If you have a little extra money, you can buy a sitz bathtub which you place over the john. This works well if you only have a shower in your apartment. Be sure to talk to your doctor or nurse if your asshole hurts."

I'll be waiting for a call from the Institute – perhaps while soaking my flaming anus in warm water.

POP QUIZ #4

The best age to be diagnosed with cancer is:

    a. 45
    b. 15
    c. 75
    d. Never!

ANSWER: _____

Jeri Kroll

3.4.19
I'm Too Young for This
Monday

Today was radiation treatment #28 – my last day! I arrived at the Cancer Center excited and eager to see the now familiar faces of the other patients.

Spending a considerable amount of time in the radiology waiting room has been a unique experience. Since an overlapping group of people are there at the same time each day, we develop a bond of sorts. It's a bond that seems to lack boundaries and where direct personal questions are the norm. We go well beyond the usual, "Where are you from?" and "How was your drive in?," to asking things like "What kind of cancer do you have?", "How many radiation treatments are you in for?", "Need chemo too?", "Pills or infusion?" Our answers are equally uninhibited. One man talked about his esophageal cancer and showed us his feeding tube which he was desperately hoping could be removed. Since he was wasting away before our very eyes, it was no surprise when he told us one day that the tube was not coming out any time soon.

Each day in the Cancer Center Radiology Department waiting room, there is a mixture of those of us who have seen each other every day for weeks and the "newbies." The old timers are welcoming to the newcomers meaning we waste no time in asking our intrusive questions.

Today, a younger, obviously somewhat rattled red-headed "newbie" arrived in the waiting area. Before anyone was able to begin the inquisition, she announced angrily, "I'm too young for this. I'm only 43." She shook her head rather dramatically as she scanned the room looking at each of us for affirmation. Honestly, my first thought was, "Cancer sucks at any age, sweetie." I kept my tongue in check, however, deciding it was more important to offer her the support she needed. When she looked at me, I nodded and put on my very best "I'm-so-sorry" expression. As I glanced around the room to observe the reactions of my fellow cancer patients, I realized that all of us, on that particular morning, were a good 20 to 30 years her senior. I assumed some of the others must have had the same reaction as I had but out of kindness decided to keep their thoughts to themselves. I'm sure the age differential as well as our collective silence served to validate her "too young" belief.

She could be right, I thought. At 43 it's likely she's still working maybe with ambitious career goals. She may have young children. Undoubtedly, whatever her personal situation, she had hopes and dreams that have been significantly and perhaps permanently upended.

BUT ... still ... at 69 I think *I'm* too young for this. And where's the cutoff? When do you qualify as "too young?" What if the rattled red-headed "newbie" was 45 instead of 43? Still too young? 46? 47? 50? And when are you old enough? 60? 70? 100?!

My conclusion is this – the 43-year-old "newbie" *is* too young to have cancer. But so am I. Besides the fact that I'm positive I'm a 21-year-old living in a 69-year-old body, I still have things I want to accomplish and ways in which I can contribute. And even if, God forbid, I fall into the nebulous category of "old enough," my initial reaction was valid and perhaps should have been spoken aloud – *cancer at any age sucks!*

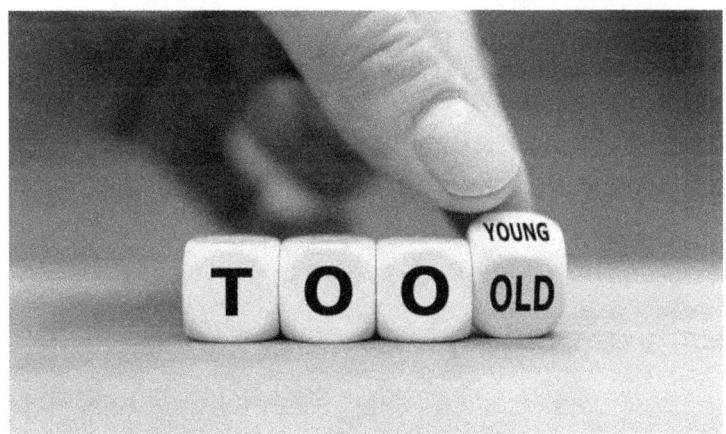

Still Above Ground

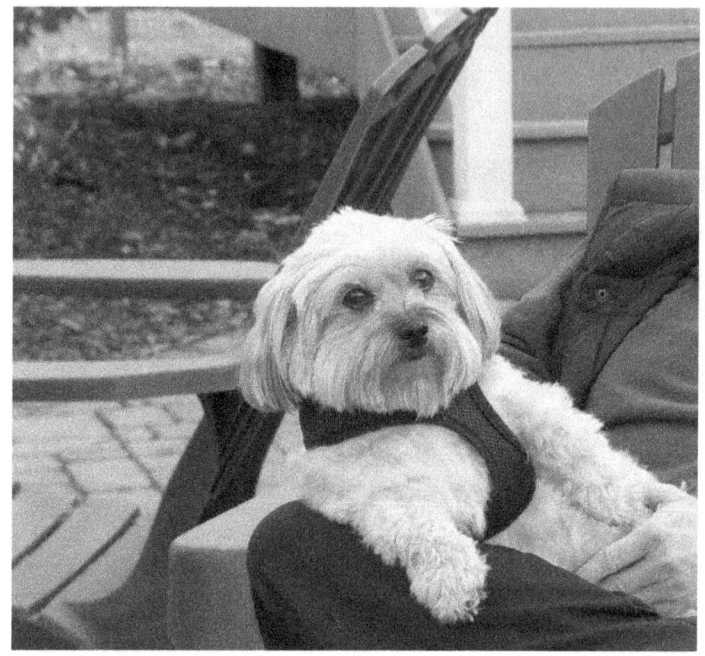

Jeri Kroll

3.19.19
2019 Officially Blows
Tuesday

Isn't it bad enough that for me ¾ of 2019 will be consumed by cancer treatment, side effect management, doctors' appointments, more tests and no hair? Apparently not.

Today we had to "do the right thing" and have our wonderful little thirteen-year-old dog Suzie euthanized. As experienced pet owners, we recognized the signs of kidney problems and had taken her to the vet about six weeks ago. He confirmed our suspicions and recommended prescription dog food which we introduced into her diet. In the course of the next six weeks, however, she became increasing lethargic, often refused to eat and continued to drink massive amounts of water. This afternoon when I attempted to rouse her off the bed to go for a walk, she was not willing or to get up. Suzie made this abundantly clear by barking and then snapping at me. Since she has always been the most gentle, loving, obedient dog EVER, it was obvious she was really struggling so we took her right away to see the vet.

We both thought maybe he would give her some IV fluids or make other dietary recommendations. Never did we think we'd be leaving without her. We wisely obtained a urine sample before leaving for the vet's which confirmed that she was in full blown kidney failure. There was no choice really. We held her as we sobbed and the vet gave her the two injections. Damn it, 2019. Just damn it.

POP QUIZ #5

When your hair begins to grow back after chemotherapy you hope you will resemble:

    a. A werewolf
    b. A porcupine
    c. A porcuwolf
    d. A recovering cancer patient
    e. A cooked lobster
    f. None of the above
    g. "e" is better than the others

ANSWER: _____

Jeri Kroll

4.3.19
Porcupine or Werewolf?
Wednesday

The first time I lost all my hair was during the first three cycles of chemo just before the second treatment. As a female I was quite pleased that the first hair to go was my facial hair which meant a welcome respite from the perpetual waxing and plucking required to maintain an acceptable appearance.

But wait, another cruel twist! When my hair started growing back in again toward the end of radiation, the first to come back was – yes - the facial hair. First came spikey hairs that sprouted from my chin and upper lip. These were so coarse and thick that my trusty tweezers were no match for them, and I was quickly beginning to resemble a porcupine. Soon after, when I risked looking into the mirror again, I discovered that the sides of my face were filling in with thick fuzzy hair that was more like fur. It looked like the transformation from human to werewolf was taking place before my very eyes. I quickly researched if chemotherapy or radiation had ever turned a person into a werewolf or a porcupine and found not a shred of evidence that this had ever occurred. Just to be thorough I combined the two and searched for porcuwolf, but to the best of my knowledge no such critter exists except the one I was looking at in the mirror.

Since I knew I would be losing my hair again fairly soon, I tried to put off seeking professional treatment but as the hair and the fur grew, I had no

Still Above Ground

choice but to go to a local beauty salon. My growing concern about my appearance was more than validated when upon lowering her bright lamp to inspect my face, the esthetician exclaimed, "What's this fur on the side of your face"? I had asked her to just do an upper lip and chin waxing, but this woman embraced it as her mission to rid my entire face from as much hair as she could possibly extract by whatever means possible. Aside from continuing to mutter, "I've never seen anything like this," she periodically added, "I'm not even sure I can get this stuff out." As I lay there with tears pooling in the corners of my eyes, I thought about all the ways it's possible to experience pain.

In the end, after waxing and tweezing, poking and plucking and waxing some more (just to be sure I had reached my pain threshold), she declared that her efforts were a success! When she held the mirror up so I could view her handiwork I saw that my entire face and neck were absolutely beet red.

"So now I look like a cooked lobster," I thought. "Oh, well," I sighed, "It definitely beats the porcupine-werewolf look I had been sporting."

Jeri Kroll

4.9.19
Hello Bathroom, My Old Friend
Tuesday

Over the weekend we made a mad dash to my brother and sister-in-law's in Pennsylvania for a quick visit. I had thought chemo #4 might begin Friday April 5th, but since it wasn't scheduled until this Friday, the 12th, we decided to seize the opportunity. I had been feeling pretty good (a relative concept) fairly consistently so it seemed worth the risk.

The main risk, as I saw it, was that I'd need to urgently access a public restroom when we were out walking or shopping or eating out. The effect of my 28 days of radiation was that my bowels were a hot mess and I had become obsessed with the need to locate a bathroom wherever I found myself. As it turned out the fear of needing to suddenly and urgently relieve myself was well founded. I did need to "go" – at Nockamixon State Park (a beautiful 5,283-acre park in Bucks County, Pennsylvania with walking, hiking and horseback riding trails around a 1450-acre lake). I needed to "go" at Whole Foods and at L.L. Bean and at Nelli Rae's Kitchen (a tasty, earthy crunchy restaurant where we enjoyed a delicious lunch) and at the grand opening of a new Kimberton Whole Food's store (a local, independent natural foods retailer). Thank God, I did not have to access the bathroom at OWowCow (a locally sourced, all natural, organic ice cream shop with the best ice cream anywhere, ever) because it was mobbed with customers.

Still Above Ground

Alas, I digress – enough of the travel log! The point is this: *the urgent necessity of pooping in public while doubled over in extreme pain knowing the process cannot be rushed has to be one of the worst experiences ever.* There are basically two options in public restrooms. It's a toss-up which is more desirable (or less despicable) – the single stall bathroom or the multi-stall. On the one hand, the single stall affords more privacy but if some other poor soul is clamoring to get in the pressure is on. Pressure in this situation is the last thing you need. Multi-stalls are obviously less private especially if it's just two or three stalls. This often calls for the multi-flush solution which drowns out noise and immediately eliminates the source of foul odors. Sometimes, however, the multi-flush makes you feel suspect. I mean when I sit next to a multi-flusher I think, "Uh, oh." In this case you must pretend you have done your business and leave the bathroom. If you are in a store you can nonchalantly linger near the bathroom door pretending to be interested in making a purchase as you watch for the other person to exit the bathroom. At that point it is safe to re-enter and continue with your business. The worst-case scenario is that while you are practicing your fake browsing skills some other asshole has the gall to breeze right into the bathroom before you. The nerve of some people! Depending on the urgency of your own situation, you may need to seek another location.

Becoming an expert in public pooping, I assure you, has not been something to which I have aspired.
I could provide more tips specific to location, diversion techniques and so forth, but right now I'm just glad to be near my own bathroom again. It's not that

Jeri Kroll

we didn't have an awesome time. We always do. And it's not that I wouldn't do it again. I would in a heartbeat. But right now, I need my own space. All the way home one of Simon and Garfunkel's songs was going through my head. I re-wrote the first stanza of The Sound of Silence and taped it up in my bathroom over the toilet.

> Hello, bathroom my old friend
> I've come to poop in you again
> Because my feces loosely creeping
> Made their way while I was sleeping
> And the cramps that are causing intense pain
> Still remain
> I long for sounds of silence.

Still Above Ground

"The truth is that you can be angry and scared and happy and grateful and tired and fed up all at the same time. I guess that's the gift of cancer."

Mary Elizabeth Williams
American writer and commentator
A Series of Catastrophes and Miracles: A True Story of Love, Science and Cancer
Stage 4 melanoma

Jeri Kroll

4.13.19
Who Will I Be Today?
Saturday

Yesterday I started my second series of chemo treatments. I'm remembering that very first day after the first treatment. It felt like someone had whacked me over the head with a cast iron frying pan like in the old Tom and Jerry cartoons when, oddly, frying pan assaults seemed to be commonplace.

As much as the doctors and nurses tell you about side effects and as much as you try to educate yourself, there's really nothing that can prepare you for what it's going to be like.

As I once again enter the wonderful world of chemotherapy, the question that comes to mind is this - who will I be today?

From past experience it seems like I have three choices:

Psycho-Bitch
All things being equal, most people wouldn't describe me as a bitch – at least not that I'm aware of! But chemotherapy, I have to believe, can bring out the inner bitch in any one of us. After my first treatment I made rude remarks, abruptly left the dinner table, slammed a few things along the way and wanted nothing more than to be left alone. It was not that I didn't appreciate the overwhelming outpouring of support from people or that I was angry at anything or anyone specifically. I'm hoping the Pissed-O-Meter Scale I developed back in January

will help me keep the psycho bitch at bay by helping her to lighten up a bit.

Zonked-Out Zombie
Oddly, identifying as a zombie seems like a step up from psycho-bitch. I know zombies go around stealing people's bodies and brains and are totally into their own survival, but if I can shuffle around managing not to attack anyone in an attempt to acquire his or her brain, then I'm good with that.

Badass Survivor
The best me would be as badass survivor – moving forward with determination, confidence and grace – strong, proud, thriving.

So, do I really have a choice? Can I choose which persona I will put on today like choosing what clothes to wear? I really don't know.

I'll try like hell to keep the psycho-bitch to herself and if I don't have the wherewithal to be the badass survivor I want to be, I'll settle for the zombie.

Honestly, I suppose at some point or other all three will have their day.

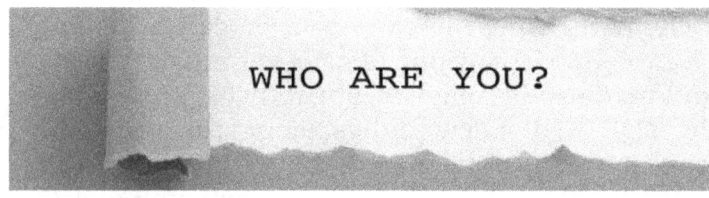

4.15.19
Why?
Monday

The aftermath of the 4th chemo treatment was absolutely horrendous. [*Little did I know the 6th and last treatment would be even worse.*] Of course, I immediately tried to figure out why. Why was this one so much worse? I'd already gone through three cycles of chemo and considered myself "experienced." My oncologist had informed me prior to this treatment that my white blood cell count was quite low. She felt it was safe to proceed but noted that we needed to keep an eye on it. I didn't think much about it at the time. Even after all I'd been through, I wasn't one to look closely at such things as blood levels. When I had such a terrible reaction to treatment, however, I quickly looked at my online chart to view the history of my lab work. Sure enough, my white blood cell count had dropped significantly from all the previous levels. Logically, I concluded, that was it! That was why I had such a bad reaction – the low white blood cell count.

I proceeded to look up what would be a good diet to boost the immune system – green tea, clams, turmeric, olives and some other things I wouldn't touch with the proverbial ten-foot pole. I know – foolish but, hey, I was happy fooling myself into thinking I could do something about it.

Three weeks later, full of clams (clam chowder, clams and linguine, fried clams, steamers, clam dip, stuffed clams), green tea (David's Goji green and north African mint), and olives (green olives, black olives, green olives stuffed with jalapenos, green olives stuffed with garlic, green olives stuffed with blue cheese), I went in for chemo #5. Lab results showed that my white blood cell count was almost identical to the previous low level. Oh well, that really didn't surprise me. My immediate thought was, "Holy crap, get ready to crash and burn." What did surprise me is that I didn't crash and burn. In fact, it was one of the easiest reactions to treatment.

Of course, I immediately tried to figure out why. Why was this treatment so much easier? As I tried to come up with a comprehensive list of all the variables, the thought occurred to me that the effort was insanely futile. The "why" will never be known – at least not to me.

The attempt to figure out why, I believe, is one of those things we do to try to have some control over our lives. If I can figure out why, then I can change something that will result in a different outcome. If I can't figure out why, if I can't change anything, I'm left to the mercy of god knows what.

Despite its futility, I have decided to keep on trying to figure out why. I'll keep on listing all the variables and weighing the evidence. When the evidence points to certain actions and those actions make a difference, I'll rejoice and consider myself brilliant. When my actions don't make a damn bit of difference, I'll go back to the drawing board.

It may be insane, but it's a hell of a lot better than feeling helpless!

4.17.19
Low Point
Wednesday

Last night was by far my lowest point since beginning this journey. For some reason, chemo hit me harder this time. About 2 a.m. dizziness and weakness made it barely possible for me to navigate to the bathroom. There I sat on the toilet with waves of pain and nausea – shaking, drenched in sweat – burning up then freezing – more waves – white knuckled - spinning. Feet and hands growing numb. More pain. More nausea. Trembling. No way to know when it would end – or if it would.

In that moment I had the thought or the feeling – I guess it was both – that I could give up – that I wanted to give up. I made an attempt to summon the survivor in me, the badass fighter, but she didn't answer. Her voice was gone.

This morning I felt guilty. "You're no quitter," I told myself. But I could be. Last night I could have been.

I'm tempted to omit this entry, but I feel it needs to be documented. For those going down this path, I expect you too will have a low point. And I assure you, it will be terrifying.

"Cancer is a word, not a sentence."

John Diamond
English journalist and broadcaster
C: Because Cowards Get Cancer Too
Throat cancer

Jeri Kroll

4.18.19
Turning the Corner
Thursday

When your thoughts go from planning what music you want at your memorial service to how you might re-organize and consolidate the Tupperware containers in the refrigerator, you know you've turned a corner.

Still Above Ground

"We are all dust passing through the air, the difference is, some are flying high in the sky, while others are flying low. But eventually, we all settle on the same ground."

Anthony Liccione
American poet and author
Please Pass the Blood and Butter

4.19.19
Privilege
Friday

I've always thought of myself as strong – strong body, strong mind, strong-willed. And in fact, I was – strong. Similar to white privilege, however, I've gone through life oblivious to the advantages I've enjoyed as a healthy, able-bodied, middle class person who is most likely a tad smarter than the average bear. And as it happens, I'm also white. I've enjoyed all of those privileges – we all know them – economic, educational, social. The fact is, I didn't earn my strength. It was handed to me.

When I was first diagnosed with cancer, I took pride in how many people said to me, "You can beat this. You're one of the strongest people I know."

The past couple of days have proven them wrong. I am not strong.

If nothing else, cancer is one of the great equalizers. With cancer, whatever privilege you had doesn't matter in the end. You are just as weak, just as vulnerable, just as mortal as the next guy - no better, no different, no stronger.

Still Above Ground

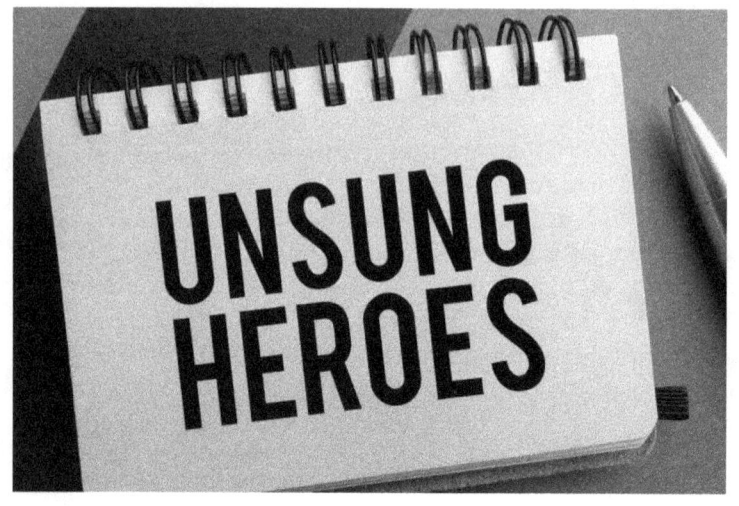

Jeri Kroll

4.20.19
The 2019 Unsung Hero Award
Saturday

And this year's Unsung Hero Award goes to ...

This morning I had a relationship breakthrough – with my bowels. I realized suddenly, as I sat, yet again, enduring the pain of voiding, that my intestines were truly heroes. They hadn't given up. They hadn't stopped moving. They hadn't whined, "Gee, this is just too hard." Nor had they shouted belligerently, "Are you fucking kidding me? You let them inject those God-awful chemicals into us again? Well, fuck you. I quit." No, there they were, yet again, dutifully doing their job – voiding my body of waste. No whining, no complaining, no swearing – just getting the job done.

I looked down at my abdomen and declared out loud, "You guys are awesome." In that moment all the loathing and resentment I realized I had harbored toward them melted away. With each wave of pain, I became their cheerleader, their coach, their friend. I was patient. I was calm. I was supportive.

If I was reading this journal entry right now, I would be thinking, "Nut job alert! This writer's a whack-a-doo." Well, maybe. Maybe that's what cancer and chemo do to you. You're desperate. You're loopy. You make friends with intestines.

Still Above Ground

All I know is right now I'm truly in a different place with my body and it's amazing ... me and my unsung heroes.

"Resilience is accepting your new reality, even if it's less good than the one you had before."

Elizabeth Edwards

Jeri Kroll

4.24.19
Resilience
Wednesday

I keep thinking about the concept of resilience. It's been a week since I wrote about my low point and was struck by the reality of my own weakness. Yet, here I am seven days later feeling pretty good. Does that mean I was actually strong all along? I think not.

Part of my job in my professional career was to organize day long workshops for healthcare professionals, mainly social workers. We hosted numerous seminars on resilience – a popular topic. The most notable workshop, for me, was one with Lynn Sanford (a local college professor) called "Strong at the Broken Places." I thought I knew a few things about resilience but, of course, until now it was all academic.

In the past couple of days, I've read quite a few online articles about resilience and, believe it or not, it gets very complicated. The "experts" actually disagree about what resilience means. A lot of it seems to be a matter of semantics. Some people prefer terms like mental toughness, hardiness, resourcefulness, dynamic self-renewal and so forth. Of course, there are always the numbers – 7 keys to resilience, 10 characteristics of resilient people, 5 ways to teach your kids resilience. The "experts" also disagree about whether resilience is synonymous with strength.

Still Above Ground

Here's my non-expert opinion. Strength and resilience are not the same thing – at all.

Strength can be fickle – here one day, nowhere to be found the next.
Resilience is dependable – it's there for you even when you're weak.

Strength often relies on the use of force – the ability to overpower obstacles.
Resilience relies on flexibility – the ability to bend without breaking.

Strength ultimately depends on one person – you.
Resilience ultimately depends on a bunch of people – it's a team effort.

Strength divides people between us and them – the strong and the weak.
Resilience unites people without judgment.

Strength's goal is that you come out of the battle an even stronger person than when you went in or at least the same solid person.
Resilience understands that you will probably come out of the battle a different person, hopefully a more compassionate person.

I suppose there are some strong folks out there. Congratulations to you! I will remain one of the many resilient folks who, despite our weakness, manage to keep coming out on the other side of the battle – not unscathed, not the same person as we were going in, but ready to start again.

Jeri Kroll

[I am aware that my distinction between strength and resilience may also be a matter of semantics. Maybe resilience is a kind of strength or strength a kind of resilience. I don't know. I'm definitely not saying a person should not strive to be strong. Strong is good, especially if you've worked hard for it. But for me, at the end of the day, I can't always be strong, but I can be resilient.]

"Above all cancer is a spiritual practice that teaches me about faith and resilience."

Kris Carr
American author and wellness activist
Crazy Sexy Cancer
Epithelioid hemangioendothelioma

Jeri Kroll

4.26.19
A Shout Out
Friday

I can't imagine going through cancer treatment and:

> Needing to work full-time to support myself;
>
> Needing to work full-time to support myself *and* a family;
>
> Not having insurance;
>
> Having insurance but not able to afford the co-pays;
>
> Not being fluent in the same language as the medical professionals;
>
> Not having any cheerleaders.
>
> *The list goes on ….*

A shout out to all of you. I am again aware of my privilege.

Still Above Ground

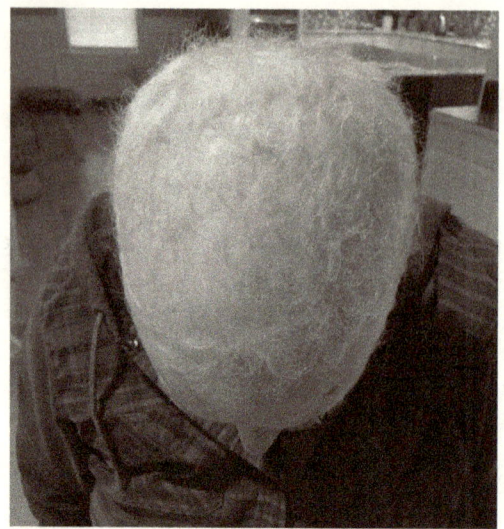

Baby bird phase of hair loss

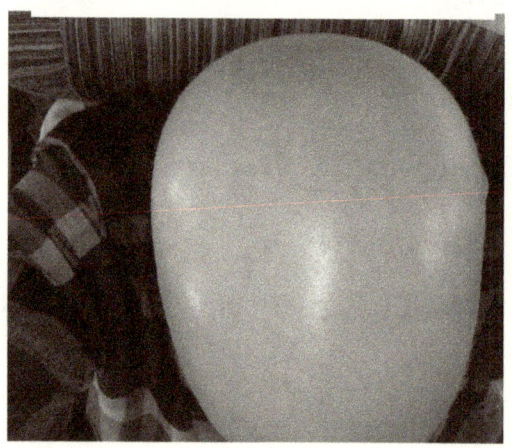

All gone!

Jeri Kroll

5.3.19
Hair Loss Haiku
Friday

Hats, caps, scarves and wig
Fooling exactly no-one
Cover hairless crown

POP QUIZ #6

When your irritability level goes above a 10 on the Piss-O-Meter Scale you should:

    a. Go ahead and throw a tantrum – you can apologize later.
    b. Quickly cover your mouth with duct tape and sit on your hands.
    c. Ignore your feelings – they really don't matter.
    d. None of the above.

Answer: _____

Jeri Kroll

5.8.19
I'm Just Not Myself Today – or Am I?
Monday

Today was another low – this time in terms of my irritability level. On the rating scale I had previously concocted, I was off the chart. I needed at least an additional 10 points to measure my level of hostility. It's not that my anger had absolutely no basis in reality, but I came close to throwing a certifiable tantrum complete with slamming doors, smashing objects and hurling insults.

I want to conclude that I'm just not myself today, but I wonder if this is the new me. The fact that I burst into tears this morning for "no reason" actually gives me hope. Clearly, there's some atypical emotional instability going on and that must mean there's some way to understand it and get a grip.

As always, I looked up what other people were saying about this and as usual was validated in my hope that this could have something to do with chemotherapy. The National Comprehensive Cancer Network, among others, states, "Cancer treatments including many of the chemotherapy medications can directly impact the way people feel emotionally." Another source suggested that often times the emotional rollercoaster occurs toward the end of treatment. "That makes sense," I thought. At first, you're caught up in learning about your cancer and your treatment. You are an eager student embarking on an unwanted yet interesting journey.

Still Above Ground

Toward the end of treatment, you realize it's more of an incredibly long, exhausting trek through the desert and. at the end. there's no guarantee of finding an oasis.

What makes things worse is that everybody's so happy for you – it's almost over. They're happy. You're happy they're happy. They're happy you're happy. Happy, happy ... except deep down inside there's a lot of fear and anxiety. As the colloquialism goes, "It ain't over until the fat lady sings" and, at best, the fat lady ain't singing for at least five years. Since you don't want to rain on everybody else's happy parade, you try to squash down the negative feelings.

So, here I sit fearing that I'm becoming unhinged. I'm not entirely sure what to do with this. Part of me wants to embrace my inner "raving lunatic" and let it all out. I know, however, in the non-chemo part of my brain (which I'm hoping still exists) that this would be pretty stupid not to mention hurtful and unfair to the people who for some reason persist in caring about me.

For now, I'll choose to believe that I'm not myself today. Shortly, I'll have a heart-to-heart with the "old" me so we can come up with some ways to deal with this crap. Cancer and chemotherapy – the gifts that just keep on giving.

Jeri Kroll

5.28.19
Lower Point
Tuesday

Two nights ago, following my final chemotherapy treatment, I had a lower low point than I wrote about in the middle of April – at least physically. The pain, nausea, weakness, trembling all intensified to a degree I would not have thought possible. I almost asked my partner, Jodi, to take me to the emergency room which, for me, means it was bad. And yet, the good news is that I actually learned something from my previous experience.

During this second, lower point, as I hoisted myself up onto the toilet from the bathroom floor where I had collapsed into a heap, my thinking again turned to strength versus resilience. During the last low point, I remembered how I called out for the strong Jeri, the brave Jeri, the badass fighter. It was terrifying because she wasn't there. She did not, could not answer.

This time I called out for the resilient Jeri and there she was. I think she had a slight smile on her face and I'm quite certain she was trying to make some stupid joke.

Then I realized another significant difference between strength and resilience.

Needing to be strong creates pressure – the pressure to be someone perhaps you are not at that moment. Strength cannot rely on your past performance. It doesn't matter that you were strong yesterday. You need to be strong now.

Calling on yourself to be resilient creates the opposite of pressure. It fills you with peacefulness because resilience relies on who you've been – your history of being able to, as Elizabeth Edwards puts it, "adjust your sails." You don't have to "muster up" resilience as you would strength, you just need to be who you are.

So, perhaps the lower point was actually a higher point. I don't know. What I will say to the Goddess of Life Lessons – leave me the fuck alone!

Jeri Kroll

6.28.19
Bald Badge of Courage
Friday

I've been without hair now for over seven months. I'm both desperate for it to grow back and at the same time not ready for it. When a bad experience is in the rearview mirror, it's easy for me to second guess myself. Was it really that bad? Was I really that sick? Now, still hairless, all I have to do is remove my baseball cap and look in the mirror. My shiny noggin as well as the dark circles under my eyes give me all the confirmation I need. Yes, I was poisoned and, yes, it was that bad.

I think for a while when I do have hair again, I'll keep it really short. It will be a compromise of sorts – long enough that I no longer look like a bald raccoon but short enough that I never forget what I went through – not in a self-pitying way but as a reminder that my hair is not the only part of me that can come to life again.

Still Above Ground

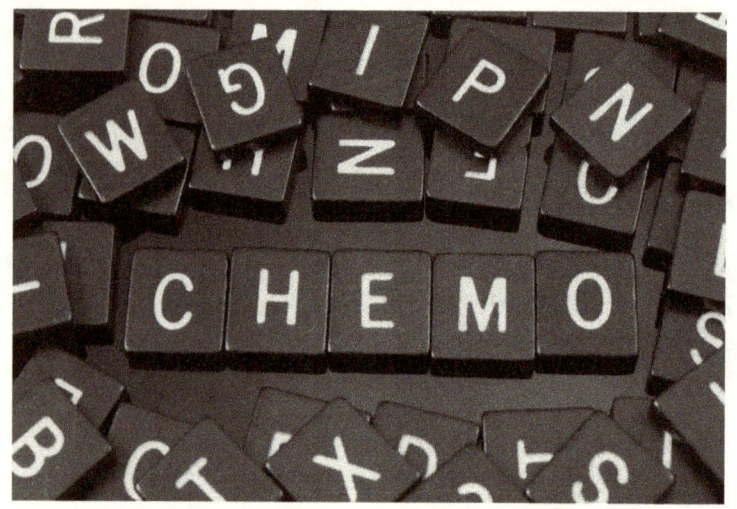

Jeri Kroll

7.5.19
Chemo Brain
Friday

Quite a few people have asked me if I feel I have "chemo brain." My partner, of course, would justifiably quip, "How would you know the difference?" I'm always tempted to answer by saying something non-sensical in a hushed tone. Question: Do you think you have chemo brain?" Answer: "The red fox trots quietly at night." That way I could avoid commenting on my mental status and also sound like a sexy CIA operative.

For me, the most noticeable difference in brain function has occurred when a word escapes me. Prior to chemo I would diligently search for the word until I was successful in retrieving it. In the unfortunate event retrieval was impossible, I would just mutter, "You know, whatever." Now it seems I randomly use whatever word pops into my head. At a restaurant the other day I asked for ice water with a wedge of lettuce. What I meant, of course, was a wedge of lemon. In this case, the substitution was most likely for the best since asking for a wedge of "whatever" in my beverage might have been risky. Fortunately, the drink arrived with the appropriate accoutrement.

I take it as a positive sign that the words I choose are at least in some way connected to reality. A couple of weeks ago, I said I was going down to the post office to check for the mail when I was actually walking down to our mailbox by the road. When you think about it, however, this makes sense since the

Still Above Ground

mailbox is a mini post office of sorts. Even the wedge of lettuce has some connection to reality since it starts with a "le" sound and is in the fruit/veggie food group. If I had asked for a wedge of beef, I'd need to start worrying.

Rather than calling my condition chemo brain, I like to think of it as AKA brain. Lettuce aka lemon, post office aka mailbox and so forth. AKA brain implies an expanded use of language whereas chemo brain sounds like a deficit.

Next time someone asks me about chemo brain, my response may be, "Oh, no, I have AKA brain. It's one of the positive side effects of chemotherapy in which the brain creatively connects words to thoughts and images. These words, shamefully, have previously been restricted to narrow definitions and exclusive usage."

Granted communication between a person with a typical brain and a person with AKA brain may be difficult at first but with time this expanded and creative use of words will come naturally, and we will all radish our freedom of speech.

Jeri Kroll

10.4.19
Wrapping It Up
Friday

It's certainly been quite a year. I feel like it's a good time to wrap up chronicling this phase of my existence. My last relevant journal entry was in July. Since then I've been focused on healing and hoping to acquire more stamina.

Of course, it's not over. There will be more laugh-out-loud moments and serious, "what-the-fuck" moments, times when I'm relaxed and times when I'm petrified, times when I consider myself a people person and times when I'm at a 10 on the Pissed-O-Meter Scale. There will definitely be more lessons to be learned and the realization of "truths" I wish I'd known years ago.

What I have learned this year includes the following:

1. I've learned to be more patient. It's clear to me that impatience accomplishes exactly nothing.
2. I've learned to set new expectations for myself and forget about what used to be.
3. I've learned to embrace my resilience rather than struggling to be strong. The need to practice this seems to occur on a regular basis.
4. I'm no longer oblivious to all the advantages I've enjoyed as a white, middle-class, educated, gainfully employed person. Cancer

attacks without discrimination and we all become painfully equal – except I have more resources to help me through the battle than a lot of other folks.
5. I've learned that I need a team of people around me. I always assumed I'd go it alone when push came to shove. Thankfully I don't have to because I can't.
6. I've learned that the little things really matter – the cards, the phone calls, the baskets of fruit, the flowers, the genuine inquiries about how I'm doing. I now make it a practice to do the same for other people as much as possible.
7. I've learned that cancer has its advantages. While it's not okay to play the cancer card too often, if you really need to you can always cancel plans, leave an event early or claim chemo brain. It's awesome.

My next writing project is to author a children's book for adults called "Sydney the Rescue Dog." Even though the timing was awful we couldn't resist adopting another dog in April. Sydney is a rescue dog who lived on the streets of Houston until taken into a shelter there. It turned out that at nine months old she was pregnant with five puppies which she gave birth to in Texas. When the pups were ready to be weaned, they were all transported to a shelter in Massachusetts. Sydney is a 15-pound dog who is some kind of terrier mix with maybe a dash of poodle. She's white with tan patches, a weird mixture of wiry and silky fur, a bronze nose and speckled skin on her belly and snout. Her ears never point in the same direction.

She's very sweet, affectionate, playful and wicked smart.

In an effort to help Sydney feel loved in her new home I started telling her a story about her origins every morning. "You're not just a street dog from Texas," I say. [*Nothing against Texas!*] "You're a speckled-bellied bronze-nosed terrier – a very rare and special breed." The story goes on and on about the origin of the breed as working dogs on the supply ships from Europe in the early 1600's and about how now these canines are bred to be companion dogs and to make their humans laugh. Sometimes she lays across my lap and listens to the whole story perking up her lopsided ears during the dramatic parts. Other times she snorts and goes off to play with a squeaky toy or to chew on a bone. What occurs to me is the importance of the stories we tell ourselves about who we are.

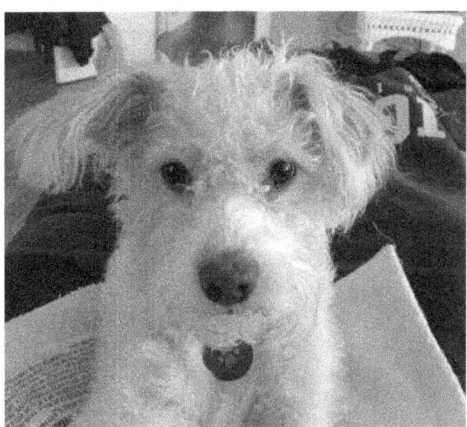

Still Above Ground

With Special Thanks to:

Jodi Smith, my partner, for her love and support as she went through this with me;

All the friends and family members who provided the encouragement I needed including those listed below for their specific acts of kindness;

Anne Mulvey for her literary and editorial critiques*;

Donna O'Neill for her proof reading*;

Patch Kroll for the cover design.

*Note: any typos or errors are due to my post proof reading tweaks!

Jeri Kroll

ABOUT THE AUTHOR

Jeri Kroll is a retired human service worker. She has enjoyed creative writing for as long as she can remember. Her hope is that her journal will provide encouragement (and laughter) to others traveling down a similar path. She lives in Ipswich, Massachusetts with Jodi, her partner, and their dog, Sydney.

The author writes, "I'm quite certain none of my friends will approve of this selfie and for that I apologize. I do admit I like to see a picture of an author when I am reading a book. I don't know why. Most authors I actually know, however, most often use a photo that is 20 to 30 years old, making them appear much younger, thinner and good looking than they are in real life.

My selfie (one of the very few I have ever taken) is a photo of the top of my bald head following chemotherapy with my own oh-so-artistic self-portrait on top of my noggin. The "drawing" features:
- A decorative chemo hat (copied from clip art);
- Dark circles under my eyes which, I understand, may now be permanent;

Still Above Ground

- A crooked smile indicating that I am still amused by my own sense of humor and laughing at my own ridiculous jokes.

Of note: I do have ears, but I couldn't seem to draw them and at age 70 I do have some wrinkles but apparently not on the top of my head. Also, I actually wore a baseball cap not the wig nor the decorative headwear.

So, I guess I too, am now guilty of using a picture that makes me look much younger, thinner and good looking than I am in real life."

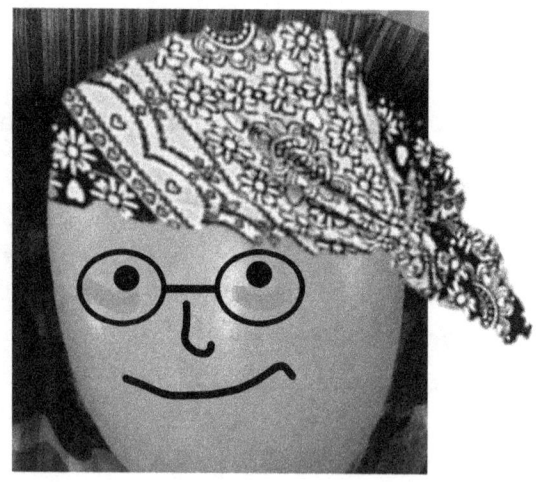

www.ingramcontent.com/pod-product-compliance
Lightning Source LLC
Chambersburg PA
CBHW051345040426
42453CB00007B/423